"Emily has a charm
making you feel like a girlfriend over for a cup of tea and a heart-to-heart. A very enjoyable read that many moms from different walks of life will find relatable and encouraging."

—CINDY MORGAN

singer/songwriter/author/wife/mother

"*For All Maternity* is like a prenatal coffee date with a best friend who's already had her baby. Emily Pardy takes readers on a witty and lighthearted journey through the early days of motherhood that will put any uptight mom-to-be or new mom at ease. Such a delightful read! "

—JESS WOLSTENHOLM

co-author of *The Pregnancy Companion* and *The Baby Companion* & co-founder of graceformoms.com

"*For All Maternity* is honest, funny, real, encouraging, and thoughtful, and is a must-read for those women who want kids, are pregnant, or like me, already have kids. Thank you, Emily for your honest transparency and your great sense of humor. This book will be an incredible resource for many women. I already have a list of friends I'll be giving a copy to."

—NATALIE GRANT

Grammy nominated, Dove Award winning
Recording Artist & author

"I'm both a woman and a mother. Emily Pardy's heart is a breath of fresh air into a world where those two things can be more than challenging."

—PLUMB

Recording Artist, Songwriter,
& author of *Need You Now, a Story of Hope*

For All Maternity

For All Maternity

What they didn't tell me about marriage, motherhood, and having a baby

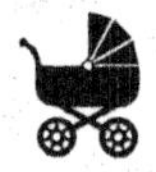

EMILY PARDY

Mountainview Books, LLC

For All Maternity

Edited by Carol Kurtz Darlington

ISBN: 978-1-941291-10-8 (paperback)
ISBN: 978-1-941291-11-5 (ebook)

Dedicated to the dads
without whom we would have no one to watch the kids while Mommy takes a coffee break to read this book. So . . . thanks, dads. Keep it up.

Special thanks to my baby daddy. Josh, I love you. I'm so grateful for you.

Table of Contents

Many Kinds of Mommies

There will be a lot of mommies out there who will be picking this book up while they are with child, given it at a shower perhaps. Or maybe a friend will pass it on after reading it themselves.

I have a huge heart for the mommies out there. I was raised by one; so were you. I became one and have forever joined a life-altering club that has a membership with no expiration. No matter what. Nothing else in this world can give you that guarantee. But if you have ever seen those two little pink lines streak across that urine-soaked piece of plastic early in the morning, you have joined the ranks of countless women who have braved the path before us. You have become a mother. Forever. And no matter who that baby becomes, how that birth goes, or to where you move on from there, you will always have the heart of a mother.

I want to say first off that I am a huge believer and supporter of adoptive moms as well. I don't want to discount you in any way. You matter. You are 100% in the club. You are 100% anointed to be rearing the child you have embraced as your own. But I want to let you know up front and honestly that at this point in my life I am not an adoptive mother, so I'm writing this from the perspective of a biologically-birthing mother's point of view. (I just hate to use the term "natural" as if adoption is "unnatural" in some way—it's not!) So I genuinely and wholeheartedly ask for your grace in reading on. I hope I never say anything that makes you feel the least bit like an outsider in the mommy club. Truly, you adoptive moms have a whole other story to tell, and while much of this book can translate, I hope that you find—or write for yourself!—another book that can speak to you exclusively and support you in your walk as an adoptive mom. All that to say, rock on. I love you. I hope you keep reading.

For those of you who are wondering who the heck I am and why in the world I'm writing this, I'll tell you. I am *you*. Seriously, no scoffing or rolling of the eyes. I see you! I am super, duper extra ordinary. No, not extraordinary. Extra. Ordinary. I have wanted to write a book for years. I have been waiting. Well, I thought I was waiting. Really, God was productively stirring me, patiently pressurizing me until I came to a slow and steady boil. And just when I couldn't take it anymore here it came, pouring out of me. Here it is, ready to serve up in pretty dishes and choke down the hard truth. I've percolated, and now I'm writing it. It is just time.

I'm ready to hijack phrases like "get real" and just lay it out simply for you from my perspective. And I'm just like you. I'm a mom, and I'm too busy for just about everything including deodorant, and while I once majored in English and flirted my way into earning my degree, I am not a therapist or a psychologist or a psychiatrist, but I'm not your mother-in-law either.

Now, we're going to start at the beginning. Well, not the *very* beginning. I have two loud children to get to bed, so let's start where it gets good and I'll take it from there. Lord help us, here we go.

1

Countdown to Babyland

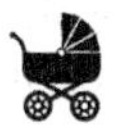

In the spring of 2008, my husband Josh and I were totally in love and ready to start a family. Or were we? Ready, I mean.

Didn't he still have student loans to pay off? And wasn't I going to lose a little more weight before succumbing my body to the burden that pregnancy was inevitably going to bear on it? Shouldn't we own a home and a dog and at least understand the basic process of the United States judicial system before entering into the realm of producing offspring? Shouldn't we travel more and see the world? Hadn't I always wanted to hole up in a cabin and write a book? Didn't he want to learn to sail a boat or at least change the oil in the car before we decided to pick out baby names together?

Then again, did you see that crib bedding at Target last week? I know, I know, I know. I shouldn't have even been looking. I would always suck my tummy in every time I entered the baby section just in case anyone should, heaven forbid, stop and converse with me and assume that yesterday's donut was an actual bun in my currently-empty oven. I always wanted to just rent a baby and take it with me for that part of the store—you know, to look like I fit in and be able to scope it out without worry or conscience—that is, conscience apart from the whole I-just-thought-about-renting-an-actual-baby notion, I mean.

Baby stuff is *cute,* y'all.

(There it is. When I get real chipper and sincere, I cannot hold back the six years I spent in the South. It. Just. Comes. Out. I don't even actually *have* a southern accent. It's just like my tongue slips into a cuteness catapult that cannot hold back. So when I see baby giraffes stretching their little polka-dotted necks up the legs of a baby's jammies in the middle of the Target baby department . . . mmm-hmmm, you can bet yer butter I'm gonna git all Paula Deen on y'all. Yummm.)

But of course giraffey-jams are *not* a reason to have a baby. Right? I mean, right. Of course not. So why do we want a baby so badly? Why do we want one now? Why don't we?

READY, SET, GO TO THERAPY

We had been married about two and a half—that half really counts at this stage—years. When we went to see a counselor our marriage wasn't in trouble. Unlike the generation before ours, we didn't believe in the notion that you had to wait until things were bad or broken in order to get yourself in front of a non-biased third party. We weren't throwing dinner plates and screaming futile insults at each other. In all honesty, we weren't even bickering beyond your normal spat of "Fine. I'll put my makeup on in the car since we're going to be late again." I mean, we *are* human here, for heaven's sake.

Indeed, the opposite was true. And so we went to therapy. We were fortunate to have found an amazing counselor a few years back when we were engaged. We both worked at a Christian university and wholeheartedly believed in building a strong foundation for marriage (hurrah!) so it was a no-brainer for us to jump into premarital counseling before saying "I do!" at the altar. Luckily, Eric (not his real name) was still at the counseling center two and a half years later when we scheduled a meeting with him to present our new dilemma of pending/possible parenthood.

I remember sitting in his office trying to control the twitching of my foot, completely giving away how nervous I truly was. And why? I had nothing to hide, really. I wasn't about to admit to an affair or a murder or a zillion other horrific ideas that this man may be licensed to encounter. I had nothing new to reveal to him that my husband didn't already know about me. I wasn't keeping any secrets and I was fairly—no, very—confident that my husband wasn't either. So, why was this twitching foot so darned difficult to settle down? And was that a butterfly in my stomach, or was I about to burp up today's lunch right in front of sweet, calm, about-to-put-my-nerves-at-ease Eric? Good grief, woman, get a hold of yourself!

He sat. He smiled. We smiled back.

It started out slow. How were we? Fine. What's new? We work here, he does this, I do that, we love each other, etc. Thank you. It was all a fine exchange. And then silence.

That's when I realized the source of my trepidation. I had no idea what to tell him! I had no drama to unfold, no tissues-for-tears sob story to break down into, no gut-wrenching turn of events to shed light on. Well, let me tell you, this happened to be the perfect setting for going to therapy.

Eric (sweet Eric) had to actually blink, look at us, pause, and say the for-real words "So, why are you here?"

Here was the best we could explain it: We were there for preparental counseling. For us, it felt like premarital counseling shouldn't stop there. We were in this back-and-forth quandary of feeling complete and then incomplete, complete couple and then incomplete without a baby . . . month to month to month.

We knew three truths about ourselves as a married couple:

1. We certainly wanted to have children at some point.
2. We wanted our union to remain unbreakable forever.
3. We wanted to see Paris before we had kids.

Since we'd been able to scratch that last one off the list just a few months before, we figured now would be a good time to ensure number two and get talking about number one. But when we started to communicate with each other about our feelings about *when* to take that leap into parenthood, we realized we were simply unequipped. And, to our surprise, we could not for the life of us find a decent book out there that would help us. Nothing at all. I mean, how hard is it to find a book entitled *Josh & Emily Pardy Should Start A Family This Summer!* Weird, right?

The thing is, unlike wedding planning where you have months of cake choosing, dress buying, flower selecting, venue staging, and in-law-greeting time to distract you from the fact that your life is going to be altered for all of eternity, making a *human being* can simply come from a single night of passion with the hubster.

One minute you're microwaving Totino's for dinner, and the next morning you wake up with a new human forming inside you. You didn't have to fill out any paperwork at the county courthouse. You have no license or expertise to ensure you are fit for this job. You haven't gotten any recommendations written up to prove to your doctor or husband or parents that you, in fact, are going to be a great mother. Nope. All parenthood really, truly takes is sex. And, well, let's admit it—we're all good at that! So we must make terrific parents, right?

Scary.

TICK, TOCK! AM I READY FOR A BABY?

We did not take this step lightly. We didn't want to just wake up pregnant and feel unprepared. Granted, many people don't get this kind of luxury! Many parents *are* stuck staring at that little pee stick with two pink lines and blinking heavily to assure themselves that this is indeed happening and is not a dream/nightmare. Many parents *have* to step up to the plate—like it or not—and, frankly put, we did not want to be those parents.

So, having the luxury of time and the illusion of control, we laid this fine, conjured-up dilemma before our counselor, Eric, as if we were the first couple in the history of marriage to be making up new reasons to go to counseling. We may be a little crazy, but we're nothing if not thorough. No one was going to sit back and blame us for not knowing what we were getting ourselves into. No, sirree.

Eric, having been solely placed in our lives by the perfect hand of God alone, was intrigued and eager. I don't think he had ever encountered such excited-to-be-vulnerable clients, and we were chomping at the bit. Of course, what he didn't know was that in the backs of our minds we were really just hoping he would say, "Oh, you fine folks? Never you mind! Parenthood is the most joyous of occasions, and you two are a perfect fit! You will make beautiful, healthy babies, and the world will surely be a better place for it. What are you two crazy lovebirds still doing here? Get outta town! Go make that baby, and don't forget to send me an announcement!"

Nope, that didn't happen. Which is why *he's* a certified counselor with many years of professional experience and schooling under his belt and my can't-wait-to-hold-a-new grandbaby-in-my-arms mother is not.

The first few sessions with Eric were fairly simple. We talked about our current life, our future goals, our presently-met expectations of marriage and work and spiritual life. We honed our communication skills and learned valuable ways to empathize and listen to each other. We reviewed our reasons for being together, renewed our focus of what we so endearingly call "Team Pardy," and reminded each other that no past, present, or future conflict would ever come between us, but rather we would approach it with a united front—not even if it came with a cute face, dimples, and pinchable little buns for us to diaper at three in the morning.

So, okay—Team Pardy is intact. We think we may want to add a new member. What's next? Time to get down to the nitty gritty.

WHEN TO START A FAMILY

It was time for us to step back, try to see the big picture, and ask ourselves a few important questions:

1. Why do we want a baby?
2. What expectations do we have in becoming parents?
3. What changes does this bring to Team Pardy?

Easier said than done. In all our talks—over dinner, after work, in bed, in the car, after church, with friends, with family, during commercials on TV, shopping for groceries, folding laundry—had it ever occurred to us to actually stop and ask ourselves these earth-shattering questions? Not really.

When the baby subject had come up it was always with much excitement—Booties! Onesies! That giant book of names!—followed by a serious look at finances and time management. Could we afford to have me stay home? Could we save money by clipping coupons? Would we be able to travel up to the mountains with our friends if we had a baby? Would they even invite us?

Granted, these are fair questions. It is certainly reasonable to know where you stand on the practical side of life before you start installing car seats only to find that your Mini is ill-equipped for a giant plastic throne that they won't let you leave the hospital without. There are specific things that *do* need to be in place to be able to jump into parenthood with relative sanity. Health insurance—or at least a means of paying for whatever birth experience you are hoping for—and a relatively secure job/paycheck are definitely worthwhile considerations. We all know this.

But I will not be the first (or last) to tell you that if we *only* consider the ledger in our checkbook or the timetable in our calendars . . . well, my friend, there simply will never come a time where your cup is overflowing with so much free time and money that you are just determined to have a baby out of sheer boredom. That's not going to happen. (And if it does, just throw this book away and go straight to therapy. You have bigger fish to fry. Please don't have a baby due to boredom.)

So we settled on the notion that we would never have enough time or money to adequately support another human life yet knowing that somehow, some way, people have been procreating for centuries on less than we had. Most of these thoughts started with "Back when our parents were our age . . ." We came to the conclusion that it was perfectly practical to start thinking we could or should broach this subject.

But we never actually stopped and hashed out *numero uno.* And now, in therapy, there it was. Out in front of us. Like the words were still floating in the sky as we looked up and then at each other, trying to form actual sentences that didn't just come out like cavemen talk of "me woman, want baby."

Why *did* we want a baby?

We were so busy asking ourselves *when* to start a family that it never even occurred to us to stop and ask *why.* After all, back before we were ever married we had already cleared the air with the whole yes-I-want-kids-someday topic. So naturally, as most dating couples do, we went straight from checking "wants kids" off the application to become my future spouse to "where are we eating out tonight?" and other super-important questions.

Wanting a baby is totally complex. I would say that the all-too-often unspoken (yet more important) debate should primarily lie in the fact that both parties just need to be on the same page. Having a variety of reasons for wanting to bring a child into the world is completely fine. Having *opposite* reasons for wanting to bring a child into the world, however, is totally devastating. That being said, if your husband is looking forward to holding a baby so he can pass on a heritage of faith and hope for a better future while you're knitting a blankie and desperately hoping to use your grandmother's middle name that's been in the family for years . . . keep talking.

Josh and I wanted a baby for a whole host of reasons. We had always wanted children as far back as we could both remember. I had twenty-seven Barbies and thirteen Cabbage Patch dolls to vouch for my childhood hopes and dreams (spoiled maybe, but still very excited at the prospect of mothering.) And my husband tells the tale of when he was very young he was asked, "What do you want to be when you grow up?" He ever-so-sweetly answered, "A daddy."

So there was one huge reason for us! We simply, innately desired to nurture a younger generation.

But there was a spiritual side to this desire for us as well. We had both recently become completely enamored with the book *A Severe Mercy* by Sheldon Vanauken. (If this is the first you are hearing about this title, please stop and make note. Text it to yourself. Google it. Find it on Amazon. Request it as a gift or buy ten copies and start a book club. Yes, it is just that good. Go ahead. Jot it down. I'll wait for you.) The book is the grand, true, heart-wrenching love story and the personal, spiritual journey of a couple seeking truth and love and knowledge. The Vanaukens became personal friends of C.S. Lewis, and they exchange many letters throughout the book.

This book had been recommended by our counselor, Eric, back when we were seeking premarital counseling. So it was kind of ironic that now, while we sat before him once more a little further along in our own journey, we brought up this book as an example of why we wanted to have children.

The Vanaukens never had children. In all their epic bliss of maintaining "springtime love" and "inloveness" with one another, they also upheld the notion that a child might offer a threat to the oneness or union their marriage dictated. This refusal of children was troubling to C.S. Lewis, and later in his life he very boldly and honestly pointed out to Sheldon that this seemed (in not so many words) quite selfish of them.

> *One flesh must not (and in the long run cannot) 'live to itself' any more than the single individual. It was not made, any more than he, to be its Own End. It was made for God and (in Him) for its neighbors—first and foremost among them the children it ought to have produced.*

Well, C.S. Lewis is not the voice of God in our home, but he's pretty darn close. And truth is truth. This was reasonable and motivating for us, to say the least. While the Vanauken love story is absolutely one of my favorites of all time, it leaves you wanting even more out of life and love, and for us that even more meant a baby.

These, along with a trail of philosophies surrounding "we want to raise children who can help make the world a better place" and other similar notions, led us into a final discussion concluding that yes, we are on the same page here. I wanted to be a mother more than I wanted any other job in the universe and just slightly less than I wanted to be his wife. He felt the same. Team Pardy forged ahead.

The second question felt more daunting.

2

Great (and not so great) Expectations

What expectations do we have in becoming parents? While I had list upon list running through my head, I could nearly hear the crickets chirping inside my husband's skull.

It really came down to one simple thing—experience!

I had been babysitting since I was about twelve years old. My first nephew was born when I was sixteen, and now I had a total of seven nieces and nephews who had run me through the gamut of auntiedom. Not only that, but over the course of the previous few years I had nannied dozens of children, including premature newborn twins *overnight*! My toes were not just a little wet. I had literally soaked up about as much experience as a gal could get without personally birthing a child on my own. I was a sopping sponge of parental information just waiting to wring myself dry on my own descendants.

My husband, on the other hand, had never changed a diaper in his life.

Side note: It is really hard for most women to admit the first fact—I mean truly admit it comes down to experience—in action and word. It is just as hard for men to admit the second. The funny thing is that you can't have one without the other.

Having established and re-established time and again these two facts in our relationship and with our counselor, I was so proud of my husband for confidently admitting he knew absolutely nothing about babies.

What Eric helped us understand, however, is that there is a big difference between learning how to care for a baby and what parenthood looks like. This took both of us by surprise.

Here I was, thinking I would simply be teaching my husband how to diaper a baby or burp a baby or bottle-feed a baby or even just explaining for the thousandth time what the heck a placenta is or a million other pregnancy-related medical terms that somehow all translated into one basic baby-unit body-part in his brain, but no. This was not what we were talking about? (Note the question mark.)

RAISING THE ROOF ON HOW YOU WERE RAISED

Maybe neither of us had ever had a baby before, but we had both had parents! And, like it or not, that is primarily what had shaped our perspective, outlook, and goals for the kind of parents we hoped to be or not to be. This wasn't something that could be learned from a baby book or even on the job. There weren't any CPR infant classes or enough hours of babysitting I could have ever taken to learn this. Nope, this was just going to take some very honest sharing and a look back on a subject we hadn't completely delved into—How were we raised?

Josh and I were both fortunate to grow up in Christian homes with loving parents who were both still married to each other. This was a huge contributor in our likeness and similarity of each other, something else we had come to find out through our time dating, getting to know one another, and in premarital counseling.

But just because we were raised in Christian homes with similar moral standards didn't mean we were parented the same way. Our parents are very different people with extremely diverse personalities and ways of doing things. And then there is *us*, two unique individuals from these different people with our own newly-shaped ideas of what worked or didn't or "I'd never do this or that" and so on.

And so, a newly-created value system became essential to set in place for our own Team Pardy if we were going to have any sense of who we were or why in the world we cared for anything at all.

Don't get me wrong—a huge chunk of this value system had already been firmly set in place prior to marriage. Again, if you haven't caught the huge drift yet, I would advise that pre-marital counseling is the place where couples can start to build the foundation of a value system. Finding out "What I Find Important and Why" allows a couple to happily, confidently, and wholeheartedly share in each others' interests, likes, and dislikes while feeling validated and understood, not compromised or resentful. If you don't feel like you're there yet, keep talking and read on. It's not about reaching a particular place in your relationship and then being done; after all, we are changing and growing individuals, so the value system will always be a process that is ongoing.

The value system for parenthood works the same way. It just focuses on "What I Find Important *in Parenting* and Why."

So how did taking a look back at how our parents raised us help us focus on what we thought would be important in parenting our own future children?

Here's a great example: birthdays.

Josh grew up in a home where birthdays were acknowledged. There was cake, a card, a simple gift that was potentially wrapped, and you usually got to choose where or what to eat for dinner that night. Josh felt happy, loved, celebrated, and never really considered wanting more or that there was even more about birthdays *to* want. Nothing wrong with that. Happy kid, happy family.

I, on the other hand, grew up in a home where if there was an excuse to throw a celebration, by golly, a celebration was thrown! Birthdays were the utmost of these events. Each year we would alternate between having a party either at home or out on the town. At home, I have memories of piñatas, giant cakes, banners, streamers, stacks of gifts, and buffets of make-your-own pizzas where my girlfriends and I would giggle our way through the night. On an out-of-the-house year, I could choose a handful of my closest friends and go to the mall and see a movie, a concert, go roller skating or to some other fabulous place followed by a fancy dinner out.

Maybe this doesn't strike you as a big deal, but that was just *birthdays*. My family also celebrated *half*-birthdays—as in yes, I'm six and a half!—and while it might be common to wake up to presents on Christmas Day, we also woke up to presents on Easter, Halloween, and even Valentine's Day.

Spoiled? You might think so. But, just like Josh, I didn't know any differently. So it came as a shock to me after I went away to college when my mom would ship me care packages full of gifts to celebrate the most mundane of occasions and my friends would look at me wide-eyed wondering if it was my birthday . . . again?

Sharing our experiences of how our families celebrated/acknowledged our birthdays in counseling became a nonvolatile plumb line for viewing our own parents' choices in raising us. It became clear to us just how gray the area of parenting could be. Sure, there are certain black-and-whites about it all—*don't* let your kid run with scissors, *do* get your kid to eat vegetables. But as we took a step back and realized how simple acknowledgements of birthdays versus grand celebratory extravaganzas were based on our parents' own value systems, we could see that there wasn't necessarily just one "right way." We both felt valued and happy on our birthdays growing up. And we both wanted that for our future kids. But recognizing that we were coming from two very different yet not wrong backgrounds, we could see the potential for a simple misunderstanding escalating into an argument over whether we would rent a Princess Bounce House for our daughter's third birthday party simply because we might not understand what the other person values.

I'll say it another way. You could lose a lot of time arguing about stupid crap that has nothing to do with what you really care about.

If we didn't take some time to think about our value system now, I could end up screaming at my husband on our baby girl's birthday, trying to convince Josh that "This is just how birthdays are done!" while he is deepening his bitterness and feeling completely misunderstood in wanting to save a buck and gritting his teeth in handing over yet another stack of bills for cupcakes that he will resent with every bite. To him, "*That* is just how birthdays are done!" Not with all the ridiculous fanfare and wasted money.

Okay, so maybe a birthday is a silly example. Maybe you are sitting there thinking, "Oh good grief, I would never yell at my husband over cupcakes or hold a grudge because of a bounce house!" Perhaps, but that's not the point. The birthday discussion was a nonvolatile topic outside of ourselves that helped us view the differences in what we valued and why. I wasn't going to take offense from him asking me questions about a hypothetical party that we weren't even throwing yet. He wasn't going to get defensive if I asked him more about his birthday memories growing up or what he wished for his future children's celebrations and whatnot. It was a great way to just get the conversation started and begin to slowly gauge our expectations of what it would look like to make decisions together for this new human we were going to be in charge of raising. Now *that* was a new idea altogether!

Something else you might be wondering: Why discuss potential arguments that haven't even happened yet? This might sound like a recipe for disaster, like we were trying to stir up drama that wasn't there or looking for a way to take a jab at each other for no reason at all. Maybe it seems scary to think about predicting confrontation or assuming one of us might react a certain way before we even give them an opportunity to step up. It might even, in extreme circumstances, appear manipulative in some way—that if one of us can nail down a decision about something now we will get our way later if the subject ever surfaces.

I get it. I hear you. I also have thought these things and wondered how it might pan out or if it would be worth it. After all, you simply *can't* predict what life will bring your way, so why even try gearing up for a future that is ultimately unknown?

I'll tell you why.

3

Truth, Traffic, and Avoiding Trouble

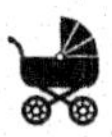

You may have never even considered going to counseling or seeking out a third party to help you and your spouse build your communication skills when things were feeling *good.* Most of us grew up with an if-it-ain't-broke-don't-fix-it mentality when it comes to marriage, so our relationships tend to dwindle somewhere between satisfactory and tolerable most of our lives. Sure, there are spurts of head-over-heels butterfly feelings for our spouse followed by the occasional I-can't-handle-how-annoying-you-are-to-me day here or there. And for the most part we skate through day to day, pay the bills, make the Costco trips, and smile when we finally go out to a movie (though sometimes it might be hard to tell if I'm smiling because of the popcorn or because I get to be out alone with my husband.) Is this the relationship you want? Is this the marriage you hoped for? Is this the life you wanted, to just "get by" and hope for a genuine smile once a weekend?

We didn't want to settle for that. And we still don't. We try to approach our marriage *preventatively.* Instead of waiting for trouble to find us and then scrounge around for skills we don't have to try and fix it, we gear up *now*, ready and aware and hopeful that we might never have to use the skills we are improving upon daily.

Really, we're talking about basic communication and sincerity (you need both.) When you are feeling in love with someone, wanting to be with them, wanting to please them and to serve them, you are more vulnerable to listen to them and be honest about who you are and what you want and need.

Remember how you felt when you first got married? You would think about him all day long. You couldn't get enough of him. And you would probably be willing to do whatever it took to just be with him forever. Well—and here is the glorious thing about marriage—*nothing has changed.* Yes, maybe you fold his underwear now and hear him fart in his sleep and can't stand the way he bites his nails when he's watching TV, but your marriage vows sealed a covenant stronger than any annoying habit could ever break. You are still willing to do whatever it takes to be with him forever. And, though he might not tell you quite as often as he once did, he most likely feels the same way about you! *This* is a good time to go to counseling.

This is a good time to predict difficult scenarios, to practice nonvolatile arguments and to protect the foundation of your marriage.

Think of preventative counseling like a vaccine. As we all know, a vaccine contains a small strain of the actual virus so that your body builds up immunity to the real illness. A tiny bit of discomfort now so that you develop a resistance and don't have to endure the real trial of the sickness later on. Preventative counseling essentially works the same way. You need to learn about yourself, about the opposite sex, about the tendencies, feelings, fears, and hopes of your spouse. You should want to learn these things (again, think back to those early days when you couldn't get enough of each other) and be willing to share them yourself. And as you communicate and dive more deeply into whom each of you is, you can begin to make sense of what your future might look like.

THE RELATIONSHIP MAP: IS THERE AN APP FOR THAT?

Most of us have smart phones these days. I use mine for everything—Facebook, recipes, email, photos, weather, you name it. And, living in Southern California, I often have to use an app for traffic. Ugh, traffic! I hate it. I will avoid it at all cost. Even if I have to take a slightly longer route, I would much rather be moving than just sitting still and waiting on others. Call me impatient, but traffic will always be on the top ten of my list of completely futile things in this life. Luckily, with the app on my phone I can glance at a map of the freeways and see where the traffic is. It shows me paths of green, yellow, and red, indicating the heaviest traffic or whether there is an accident up ahead. When I'm in a time crunch, this map can save me hours by avoiding huge obstacles ahead. I might end up taking a road I never have been on before. I might see something new I didn't know was even in that neighborhood. I might learn a faster or more convenient route I never would have taken otherwise. But I'm always glad I used the app by the time I reach my destination. I'm always thankful I'm not *still* in traffic, or worse, *in* the accident that was blinking bright red on the map.

Unfortunately, our smart phones don't have an app for relationship accidents. Those are a little harder to predict. But if you could look at a map of your future with your spouse and see where those blinking red lights are, would you want to avoid those routes? Would you take another path, even if it were a little longer? Yes.

Sometimes the scenic route is not only more beautiful, but safer as well.

4

How in the World Do I Know I'm Ready to Start a Family?

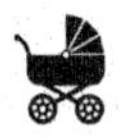

It was in our own preventative counseling that we were determining our newly-formed value system for Team Pardy. What did we truly *value*? What did we want to pass down to our children and why? Before we could get into specifics like "what size birthday party are you expecting for our yet-to-be-conceived youngsters?" we had to get a better grasp on what Team Pardy was really working towards.

For us, it came down to three things. Mind you, these are not original thoughts. We are not the first (I don't know who is, honestly) to come up with some points for what we want out of life. And it's not like our home looks like a board room with these things on an overhead projector reminding us via PowerPoint the priority list of how decisions are made in our home. Good heavens, these points are not to bring rigidity to the relationship. They are simply to help us envision and align our decisions with what will actually help us achieve our hopes and dreams! That being said, here is what Team Pardy values, in particular order:

1. Holiness
2. Healthiness
3. Happiness

Simple enough! (See? That was much less painful than you anticipated, wasn't it? It's okay; you can admit it. I know I was starting to get all "therapist" on you, and you were worried someone might mistake you for reading a self-help book there for a moment. Never you fear!) Remember, this isn't "what's right" necessarily. Each couple's value system is dependent only upon *what they value most*, so don't just steal the Team Pardy Value System and slap your name on it. Take the time to evaluate what you want out of life and then prioritize a few simple umbrellas that encompass your efforts towards getting there. These just happen to dictate how we lay out decision making in our home.

If the umbrella words are accurate and general enough, you should be able to use them with just about any major decision. It's not like you need to use them to address *every* decision. Most daily decisions—doing laundry, what to eat for dinner, where to buy gas, what movie to see—settle around the happiness value and don't have much further effect on others. Even if a decision is expensive, it's not like you are really worried about your health when you are picking out a new couch. If, however, you don't have the money to buy said new couch, it might not be a step towards holiness (i.e. does going further into debt for this couch fit with being more like Jesus or not?) and it's always good to reevaluate what we might not necessarily need. So in some cases, while one value might not seemingly apply, the overarching value (we value holiness *over* healthiness or happiness) trumps the others. We can trust this system since we also trust that pursuing holiness actually achieves ultimate healthiness and happiness. You get it.

It is important to note, however, that there is a genuine reason we put happiness last. Happiness is not the point to this life. And neither is healthiness. Both of those things will waver, come and go without prediction, change according to what we feel may or may not make us healthy or happy. But, holiness is rock solid. I'll admit the word *holy* conjures up uncomfortable feelings of self-righteousness in my gut. It makes me think of *holier than thou* and all those other sayings that reflect a haughty and selfish attitude. So I want to be clear that it is not pursuing a better-than-others perspective. Rather, it is *beyond* us to pursue holiness. It is not about us at all. It's about Jesus, all about Jesus. The word *holiness* then is the ultimate value of simply wanting to live a life worthy of being a follower of Christ and pursuing what *He* values. If this didn't come first on our list, nothing else on the list would matter at all.

This is the system we could then apply to our grand question of parenthood, to the one mystery still looming in our hearts—when should we start a family? Since our value system was intact, we could take this question and filter it through our new lens that allowed both of us to feel validated and understood.

1. Would it bring us happiness to start a family now?

Yes. We were excited. The topic was starting to take over most of our conversations and to build up an eagerness in our hearts that neither of us wanted to end. We would see other couples with babies or hear news of someone expecting and it became our first response to feel joy and jealousy all at the same time. News of having our own baby would certainly bring happiness.

2. Would it bring healthiness to start a family now?

Yes. Physically, we were both in good shape. I had been to the doctor and had the green light to become pregnant. All systems were go, and there was no reason to think we wouldn't be able to conceive within a year, most likely sooner. We had good health insurance and a two-bedroom apartment, and while we weren't exactly sure how to afford the baby once it arrived—the question of would I still work or stay home had yet to be determined—we knew that our jobs were secure and that we had plenty of areas to cut back on if need be. (Did we really need the sports package on our cable? Did we really need to get Starbucks *every* day?) We were in a reasonable and healthy place to allow for another being to thrive under our supervision.

3. Would it pursue holiness to start a family now?

This, of course, was the ultimate question. It was as if we were asking, "God, do You want us to have a child now?" Which is exactly what we had been praying the last several months. Certainly it was within the realm of pursuing a Christ-like life to want to have a baby. Time and again, the Bible reminds us that children are a blessing and to be loved and cared for as we are loved and cared for by God Himself.

It was at this question, also, that we had to succumb to a new and nearly debilitating reality—this was out of our hands. If we could decide that it would bring us holiness, healthiness, and happiness to have a child now, all the decisions on our end were made. We were going to go for it.

The rest was up to God.

5

Storks and High Stakes: Time to Take the Plunge!

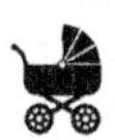

We were about to become parents. Or at least it felt that way. As soon as we made the decision to open that door and officially "start trying," it felt like I woke up every morning with a new symptom making me believe I was pregnant. Every time we had sex that first month, no matter how passionate or spontaneous, a new fear and giddiness would sweep over us (more fear for him, giddiness for me) that we might have just created a human being. The wonder and freakiness of it all was simply bewildering.

Still in counseling, we would gauge our expectations, trying to be honest about the excitement and additional purpose our intimate life had taken on. I had a friend at the time reveal to me that she and her husband were going to start trying this same month as well. Three weeks later, she was making the big announcement—they were pregnant! She was ecstatic, and I was thrilled for her. Not only for her, but to be honest, her quick success at pregnancy (yes, their first try!) gave me unrealistic hope in thinking I too could be celebrating a pregnancy within the week. It even sent a sense of competition running through my ovaries. *C'mon body, if she can do it, we can do it!*

We told Eric that we were not holding our breath this month but trying to be realistic that it would most likely take about three months to get pregnant. This seemed reasonable. It was May, and looking to the end of the summer seemed far enough away. Certainly we would be registering at Babies R Us by October and having baby showers by Christmas. Yes, that calendar looked good to us.

"And what if it takes longer?" Eric asked us both.

I don't know if I said it out loud at the time or not, but I remember immediately thinking, "Why would it take longer?" Three months already seemed like an eternity to wait for something we'd been hemming and hawing over for months already. We'd decided we were ready for this. We were making enough love to conceive an army. We were healthy and happy and my work schedule was lighter in the summer, which would be perfect timing to start adding in doctor appointments. Why would it take longer? Why? Why?

We didn't have an answer to this. We just didn't know how long it would take. And planning for the unpredictable was something entirely new for my type-A system to attempt to process.

WHY CAN'T WE TRACK STORK FLIGHT PLANS?

We were not pregnant that first month. While we told ourselves this was within our reasonable expectations, the truth was that my friend's belly was starting to grow and mine was empty. My period had been ten days late—for no reason but to cruelly trick me into holding out hope (and pee sticks.) The truth was we had held our breath after all, and the exhale was painful. But it *had* only been one month. Okay, we were going to have to pace ourselves.

Eric could see our disappointment. He was watching us enter into uncharted territory and already feel up against a wall. So he gave us an idea that truly set us off on the right foot. "Why don't you celebrate your couplehood before you take the step into parenthood?" he said. "Not just celebrate your couplehood, but grieve it too. This is the end of a chapter and potentially the beginning of a new one any day now. What better reason to stop and look at what you have right now?"

Now, *there* was an idea.

Grieving our couplehood. No one had ever mentioned anything like this before. None of our friends who were parents ever said anything about not being a couple anymore. Sure, they would mention/complain how hard it was to get alone time. They would tell us how we should sleep more, see more movies, travel while we were still free. But they never said anything about how they would miss those days of not having children, of life being just the two of them. Maybe it would feel too honest—wrong even—for them to say that once in a while they longed for the time before 3 a.m. feedings and diaper blow-outs. Secretly, were they feeling guilty for missing those days? Were they wishing they had not taken their freedom for granted when they had it? It's hard to say. It seemed quite understandable to us.

Yes, we were excited and ready to change our lives with a baby. We were eager to embark on the new chapter of parenthood. But there would be several things we would miss about our current life, and we wanted to be honest about that. After all, this was not our first life change. We had stepped out of singlehood and into couplehood not so long ago when we were married. And each of us could relate to that kind of change— change for the better, but still change. Surely, stepping into parenthood would be a similar kind of alteration.

That was as familiar an experience as we could relate to. When we were single, it was true that we could literally do anything we wanted whenever, however, and wherever we wanted without any obligation or consideration of another person. But we had spent most of our single adulthood yearning to find each other. We desired someone to share our life with, to love and consider till death do we part. And when we finally found each other and knew it was forever, we sealed that deal and never looked back. There are two essential differences between these stages of life, jumping from singlehood to couplehood compared to jumping from couplehood to parenthood.

First of all, you get to *choose* your spouse. You search and search and pray and date and pray some more, and months of drama later . . . *voila!* You have sent a boy head over heels for you and he has popped the question and your girlfriends are buying you lingerie and everyone is sending you cards with money inside. It's a magical time, really. And, for the most part, with lots of good discussion (and quality premarital counseling) you know whom you are choosing to spend the rest of your life with.

Not so with a baby. You don't know who this human being is whom you are potentially creating every time you sleep with your spouse. You have hopes and dreams that this baby will be the perfect combination of all your best qualities. He'll have his father's eyes and his mother's gentle spirit. She'll have her mommy's smile and her daddy's wit. He'll want to build tree houses with Daddy, and she'll be a perfect sidekick in the kitchen with Mom. But there's just no guarantee. Your baby could be colicky and up till 4 a.m. for the first eight months. Your baby could be sick or need special care or learn differently than others. Your baby could be premature or come very late or might cry all the time or might be calm all the time or might not nurse well or might need more food than you can provide or might not travel well or might not take a pacifier or maybe won't look anything like either of you. Heaven forbid, your baby might be ugly and everyone will stare and tell you how much she looks like your hairy Uncle Ned. (Deep breath, deep breath.) The point being, you don't get to choose your baby.

Secondly, you are in charge of scheduling your own life. Even when you are a couple, you dictate your plans and usually the woman schedules the events of the day/week/month and the husband is commonly secure and happy to oblige. They tend to not want to hold the calendar anyway. In fact, most husbands are thrilled to give up that part of their singlehood so that the wife can now just tell him where to show up and what to wear so they can know what to do with themselves each night. (A blanket statement, maybe, but generally the case.)

From the moment the Save-the-Date cards are sent out for your wedding day, you feel a sense that, yes, this is all right on schedule with your life. No matter how old you are or how long you waited for your wedding day, when it finally arrives you look back and feel a sense that certainly it came right when it needed to. It was worth the wait, the effort, the money, and it just so happens that if such and such hadn't occurred right then—blah, blah, blah—this day might never have happened. (We know this because that story is told in every speech at every wedding reception for every couple.)

Babies don't have calendars. The truth is there is just no telling when you might get pregnant, when that baby might arrive, or when this new, life-altering stage of life will show up. If only we could track the flight plans of storks and predict when one might land on our doorstep, swaddled bundle of joy in tow!

Not knowing the future, not knowing when our couplehood would be up and this new stage of our life begun, we set a time to grieve. This might sound terribly dark to you. Maybe you are picturing a couple dressed in black, crying and holding each other and wondering why in the world we are coming up with new reasons to focus on loss. Please don't jump to conclusions; it was nothing like that. This grieving process was a time to celebrate!

We got a room (bow-chicka-wow-wow) at the hotel where we went directly after our wedding reception. It was local, so it didn't cost us an arm and a leg, but it was far enough away to feel like a genuine escape from our daily life. We figured if we were going to truly grieve our couplehood wholeheartedly, we might as well also get a head start on our parenthood too. Besides, several couples had told us that it was when they got away that they felt stress-free and were able to conceive, so why not give it a go? We went to a lovely place for dinner. We watched movies in bed and stayed up late talking. We slept in and had too many waffles for breakfast. We indulged in our lack of schedule and total freedom. And we sat across from each other and just stared, like we used to do before there were rings on our fingers and bills in both our names and rent to pay and work to do. The world faded away and there was just us, only us, to enjoy and behold. We were going to miss this. We were forcing ourselves to miss this. We were staring at each other, taking it all in, intentionally feeling the gratitude and weight of each second ticking by. This memory was going to be burned into our brains, so help us. We would always remember that this family—no matter how big it might grow to be—started here, with *us* and our combined hopes, fears, and love for one another. That our children—real, actual human beings!—would spring from the making of love itself. Awesome.

And then we went home. Maybe on the outside nothing had changed. We still weren't pregnant (that we knew of) and our daily life remained the same. But something had changed in us. The weekend away had brought an entirely new sense of closure and purpose to our lives. Grieving our couplehood had granted us a new perspective on how precious these days were together. It felt like we had given our new chapter a proper celebration, just as we had done with our wedding when we entered into couplehood from our single lives. It felt new, exciting, and very, very intentional. The moment had been marked on our hearts, if not our calendars, and we welcomed the emotional roller coaster that was ahead of us. Little did we know just how long that ride would last.

6

When Trying Feels More Like Failing

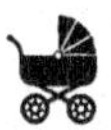

Our counseling gave us a chance to step outside of ourselves and see our life together as something greater than just two people trying to get along. We had new tools in our relationship toolbox, we had new skills at the ready, and we had new motivation to give of ourselves more vulnerably and completely than we had before. It was a natural and satisfying closure as we shared our thanks and said our good-byes to Eric when he moved out of state, looking forward to sending him a baby Pardy birth announcement in the not-too-distant future.

HUSH ABOUT LITTLE BABY?

We were a few months into "officially trying" when we realized that nobody else around us really knew about this exciting new phase of our life together. Surely, it would come as no surprise. It was widely known that we looked forward to parenthood "someday" and that we had an empty second bedroom in our apartment that just sat there begging for a purpose to be decorated. Still, the days went by and we felt like secret spies on a covert mission. Our marriage had a new purpose under its belt, and no one was the wiser to it. I might be pregnant *right this very second* and nobody would have any idea. We might have just formed a new life inside my body, and not a soul could tell by looking at me. It was all very weird.

We went to work like normal. We got up and did laundry and dishes and watched TV every night before bed just like the night before and the night before that and so on. And finally, for some reason, one day we just couldn't take the pressure of it any more. We had to tell someone!

This gave way to the discussion of the "inner circle." Who would we tell? Up until that moment, we had felt like we shouldn't say anything until we actually had something *to* tell. But this was an exciting time, and it came with mountains of emotion that we wanted to share.

The decision to tell others you are trying to get pregnant is different for each and every couple. There is no right or wrong way to do it. There is no better or worse time to share it. The only thing that is the same for everyone who decides to let the cat out of the bag is this—once you say it, you can't take it back. We needed to be selective in who we told. Opening this door was also going to open up the opportunity for others to speak into our very intimate, very up-until-now-completely-private life. People aren't going to high-five you and hand you lingerie like at your bridal shower. People aren't going to just smile and pray for you silently. Telling people you are trying to get pregnant means that every time this person looks at you from now until the big announcement they are going to glance at your belly and wonder if you are with child. It means that when they ask how you are they really mean, "Should the booties I'm knitting for your baby be pink or blue?" It means that every time you say something like "Well . . ." or "So . . ." or any other kind of pause after just about any word, those friends are going to raise their eyebrows in anticipation of celebrating a pregnancy announcement. Which sounds like a great thing until you end your sentence with " . . . I'd better get back to work" or " . . . See you tomorrow" and their faces drop with disappointment again.

We needed support, not pressure. We needed hugs, not

advice. We needed love, not lectures. So the inner circle became a very selective group of close friends and family who would pray for us and our new leap towards parenthood. Our criteria for choosing whom we told was important but not lengthy. It was fairly simple, really. We just asked ourselves, "If we encountered loss, who would we call on?" This group of "in the know" friends became the same individuals who made the cut for people we would be the first to tell once we saw those two pink lines on a pregnancy test. If only we *could* see those two lines show up on the pregnancy test.

CAN I STRANGLE MY OB/GYN?

Eight months into trying, I was officially pissed off and worried. This was the longest anyone in my family had ever taken to conceive a baby, and the thought that there might be something wrong with me started to intrude into my brain. I made an appointment to see my gynecologist. It had been about a year since my last appointment anyway, so I figured it was worth a visit.

Everything was normal. Everything looked good. You would think this would bring a sense of relief (of course it did to a certain degree) but part of me was disappointed. I wanted a reason. I wanted a baby and I didn't have one yet . . . without explanation. I sat in the doctor's office, uncomfortably shifting my bare butt on that annoying, crinkly tissue paper that covers the examination table and quizzed my doctor left and right. I wanted to know everything there was to know about conception. I had done my homework on ovulation, cervical fluid, basal body temperatures, early pregnancy signs, and so forth. I had charted my cycles and kept a journal of my symptoms. I'd been certain all my efforts must be leading to the perfect baby being conceived any day now if the doctor would just give me a magic pill, or at the very least, some encouragement to try such and such and send me on my way with renewed hope.

Instead, my doctor scribbled something on my chart and said, "Eight months isn't really that long. Don't worry."

Not that long? This was the last thing I wanted to hear. I had not anticipated leaving the doctor's office feeling completely invalidated. Disappointed maybe, but invalidated? I wanted to strangle her. Eight months *is* a long time. Eight *days* is a long time when you want something and can't have it. Eight *minutes* was starting to feel unbearable, and here I was being told that all my worries and stress and effort toward making something happen were really not that important after all. I was furious. And hurt. I felt entirely helpless.

For the last eight months (and who knows how many more were to come) I had lived my life two weeks at a time. The thing about trying to get pregnant is that your thoughts, feelings, and emotions are constantly on hold, constantly scrutinized, and constantly changing moment by moment. For two weeks of the month you are optimistic, motivated, and confident that *this* will be the day a new life is made. You have fun, you have purpose, and you try to keep the attitude light and the bedroom romantic. After all, you want this special moment to stem from love, not agenda.

The next two weeks you wait. This is aptly called "the two-week wait" (TWW) for all those ladies out there "trying to conceive" (TTC.) Yes, there is a shorthand language the internet community has invented just for us! You wait and wait, and you swear that every little thing you think or do or say or see somehow affects the possibility that you may or may not be carrying a child.

Was that a tugging sensation near my right ovary? Was it more of a tugging or a sharper, jabbing pain? Could that be ovulation? Did I miss the window or calculate incorrectly this month? Or is it implantation? Is the embryo trying to attach itself right at this very moment? Is that even something you can feel? Am I the first woman ever to be able to feel that because I love this baby more than any person has ever loved a baby before?

Every trip to the bathroom becomes a potential surprise party. This sounds ridiculous, but it's true. You've never even thought about examining your Underoos before, and now it is the difference between baby and no baby.

Is that pink? Am I starting my period? Do I feel crampy, or is it a different feeling than last month? Does my pee smell weird or did I just drink too much coffee this morning? Is that even a symptom? I do feel a little nauseous; could it be morning sickness? Should I test again when I get home? AM I PREGNANT?

And then you test. You test and test and test and test. You pee on so many sticks so many mornings that you can't even remember the last time you went to the bathroom just because your bladder was full. You read the instructions on the box again and again and again just to be sure you didn't do it wrong (even though there really is only one way to pee on the darn thing and by now you could practically enter the Olympics in stick-peeing and come out with a gold medal.) You count and recount the days since your last potential date of conception and count and recount forward to the latest possible date your period might show up. And every time you see it—one more negative test—it feels like someone punched you in the stomach.

And then your period arrives. Devastation sets in, and you drown your sorrows in a glass of wine that you otherwise had secretly hoped never to be able to consume again (well, not for the next nine months at least.)

Each month the roller coaster takes a new and unexpected turn. Some months, the negative test leads to tears and anger. Others end with a shrug and that glass of wine I mentioned earlier. But for me, disappointment always remained. Without fail, the weeks leading up to the negative test would hold excitement and total anticipation of happiness. We forced ourselves to ride this roller coaster to its fullest extent, keeping our eyes open all the while. We celebrated the highs—"I think I might be pregnant! I totally feel nauseous this morning!" We suffered the lows—"This is not fair! I hate this! I can't wait any longer. I want a baby now! Why isn't God giving us a baby now?"

And it was a battle each and every month to not let myself slip into the worst emotion of all—jealousy.

7

Facing the Green Monster

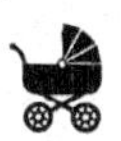

It's a cruel joke and no exaggeration to say that when you finally decide wholeheartedly to pursue something you start to see it everywhere. The entire world seemed pregnant except for me. Anywhere I turned I ran into strollers, bumped into babies, and knocked into protruding pregnant bellies. It was like, in all my effort to conceive, I had somehow developed a special radar system able to spot a baby bump from a mile away. Strangers, neighbors, and close friends were all popping up pregnant, month after month. Some were surprises, some had been a long time coming, but all were announced with explosive enthusiasm in a grand spectacle just short of a small-town parade. At least, that is how it felt to me.

With each new pregnancy that was announced I felt like one more of my own eggs just dried up inside me. *She won this month and I lost again. She gets a baby; I don't. She has new life in her, and I'm harboring nothing but envy.*

ENVY AND HORMONES DON'T MIX

I distinctly recall one day when I was walking to my car after work. It had been a particularly exhausting day and all I wanted was to curl up on my couch with a jar of peanut butter, a spoon, and a rerun of Frasier (my go-to TV therapy) when I spotted her—a beautifully pregnant stranger, belly in full blossom, waddling to her car in all her knocked-up glory. I had never met her and didn't recognize her at all. Poor soul was probably some lovely wife of a faculty member who most likely taught a Bible class of sorts, I'm sure. Nevertheless, lovely as she was, I couldn't take it anymore. Salt water started to well up in my eyes, rage clenched the air from my throat, bitterness crippled my hands into useless claws, and in one purely horrific moment of self, I silently spewed the only words that felt familiar to me in that moment: *I hate you.*

I felt like my entire insides had rotted out and failed me to the core. All my joy and hope in conceiving the next great miracle from God had been replaced by ugly, controlling selfishness, anger, and jealousy. Of course, I didn't really hate *her.* I didn't even know the sweet gal, bless her heart, who was surely gestating what I can only imagine to be the next Billy Graham in her bulging belly. I'm so sorry, dear woman, for pegging you as my target for hatred that day. But, you should know, it was not in vain.

That moment of disgusting self-loathing opened my eyes to a vital understanding—I had no control. This sounds simple, like something as obvious as gravity. But, like gravity, sometimes it takes an apple (or in my case a pregnant lady) hitting you in the head to accept it as reality and see how it really applies to your life.

I remember trying to convey these revolting feelings of jealousy to my husband. I was having a hard time relaying the significance and the sheer toll they took on my daily mental state. I kept saying the same things over and over again with nothing but his helpless, compassionate, and completely-confused face staring back at me in total frustration. Finally, after weeks (maybe months) of weighing him down with lessons from my psyche, I found an analogy that hit home with him—something he could genuinely relate to in equal reaction.

I feel like I'm applying for my dream job every month. I have read the job description a million times and tweaked my resume to fit the exact requirements. I have extraordinary experience, outstanding special skills, unmatched training, and remarkable references. I've done everything right. Everybody thinks I should get this job. I'm well liked, wholly supported, and overly qualified. And every month, every week, every day I find out again and again that I was overlooked and someone else was chosen for the position.

This cut through the wall of emotions that had built up between us. Josh, like many men, could relate to the feeling of inadequacy in a work setting and the immense insecurity those emotions brought with it. Nobody likes feeling inferior, invalidated, or ignored. While he had been riding this roller coaster by my side, it wasn't until this breakthrough moment for us both that we felt like we were really on the same emotional page, understanding and feeling understood. What it felt like to be sad. What it felt like to be alone. What it felt like to fail. There had to be something fruitful to this miserable journey.

I had been living under the *illusion* of control. Counting days, charting numbers, calculating possibilities, and conjuring up multiple justifications for each and every potential scenario that could present itself. I couldn't help but feel that if I could just figure out what I had done or not done in the month prior I could fix it and find myself pregnant in the next round. My head knew it was by God's hand alone that a baby would be created, but my heart's habits died hard. My heart knew what it longed for, what was at stake, and what was being risked each month—the possibility that I might not get what I wanted most.

It wasn't necessarily that my actions had to change (though a mental break from tracking cervical mucus was a welcome vacation for my sanity.) My perception of what I was pursuing and how it so deeply affected me on a daily basis needed a major adjustment. I had delicately fallen into a trap of thinking that if I did A + B, then naturally C would occur. Because that's how it *should* go. Because that's *normal.* Because that's what I *deserve.*

And then it hit me. I wasn't just questioning my emotions here. I was questioning God. The illusion of control had led me along a path where I was left staring down an unknown road with a pretend map I had drawn with a broken compass. *What if I'm never pregnant? What if I don't get the future I want?* Which, if we are really being honest here, is essentially asking the real question *Do I believe God is truly good?*

That might be hard to admit. Questioning God's goodness sounds like a huge leap from asking Him when I can start registering for bottles and bassinets. But if the goodness of my future hinged on the notion that I bore a child or not, and I believed God only wanted what was good and best for my future, I couldn't have it both ways. Was I really choosing between having a baby and believing God? Certainly not. I had spent too many hours praying about my desire for a family for God to ignore the request. God knew me. God loved me. God understood that this longing in my being also encompassed a pursuit of His will for my life. So if God was good and it was good for me to want to become a mother, where was my baby?

It was time to relinquish control. This is kind of an oxymoron, really. The control was never really in my grasp to begin with. My future *is* mine, and it *is* affected by the decisions and consequences of my actions, but there comes a time when you have to face your relationship with your Creator and allow Him to function *through* you instead of just around you. God doesn't need us, after all. He is perfect and complete and entirely capable (this would be the "omni" part of Him) without our hot-mess-of-a-human existence meddling about in this crazy world He built. But He is a gracious God who engages with us, works through us, and allows us the incredible opportunity to lay down ourselves and pursue a plan worthy of His glory.

As the saying goes, I "let go and let God" take over.

Maybe not much changed on the outside. I doubt even our inner circle recognized a change in my demeanor (except maybe that I cringed a bit less when a pregnant lady was present.) But on the inside I was transformed. My prayers stopped being about ovulation and started being about peace. I stopped obsessing about my basal body temperature and started dreaming about the hopeful future of how God would shape us into parents, even if it hadn't exactly gone how we thought it might go. My heart had gone from eager to rigid to numb and was now thawing to the idea that God's best was worth waiting for and my timeline was just that—mine. I felt the raw and honest reality that truly I wanted nothing to do with me. If I was prepping to be a parent, to take on the task of somehow raising a child of God as my very own, then certainly I was in need of much more Jesus and much less Emily with every minute He made me wait.

This period of waiting didn't seem unbearable anymore like it had in the past. As I sat still in acceptance and peace I suddenly felt the most active of all the months of trying so far. It wasn't easy. It wasn't even fun. As terrible as it is, the futile actions I had become accustomed to while living under the illusion of control had brought me frantic joy, allowing me to think that I was actively participating in the creation of something that was beyond my efforts in reality. But living in the moment of relinquished control brought me unfathomable relief like I hadn't felt since before we ever uttered the word *baby*.

You might be getting your fair share of people saying, "Get away from it all and de-stress! Stop *trying* and just leave the window open and see what happens! Don't worry about it so much, and when you two finally relax it will happen!" This is just the tip of the unsolicited iceberg when it comes to advice from those around you. Honestly, I found there are only two responses to this load of crap: *Thank you* or *Shut up*. Depending on whether you'd like to keep said unsolicited advisor in your life or not, you can choose your response accordingly.

Living in the moment of relinquished control was not defeat for me, just as it was not another superstitious attempt at trying without really trying either. It was a necessary, ongoing process for my heart to weather so that I could one day look back and give credit where credit was due—God's goodness. God's grace. God's creation. God alone.

I still didn't have an answer as to why God was "making me wait." But I rested wholly in the security of knowing that God knew, and God's goodness justified His reasons, and Him being God and all pretty much summed up any other questions

I had for Him and His lack of sharing his Google calendar with me (assuming God uses Google.) I wasn't avoiding the stress of trying to conceive a baby. I was giving it to God instead. (Can we all take a collective deep sigh of relief? Ahhhh.)

But sitting still and actively waiting are two different things. And they are not mutually exclusive.

8

Peace, Pins, and The Best Plans I Never Made

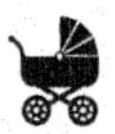

While my actions had changed as a result of relinquishing control, my passion for a child didn't diminish. In the ebb and flow of my "trying" I had to come to terms with what else might be a possibility to pursue in an effort to help our chances. In other words, taking action or certain steps toward your goal does not negate the need for God's ultimate feat. Life is *His* miracle. He alone creates.

It was with this new peace, new outlook, new hope that I cautiously took the next step. I called my doctor and made an appointment for fertility testing. It was a couple months away, as they don't diagnose you as infertile until after you have actively tried to conceive for at least a year, but I needed the date on the calendar to help me pray through and cope with the notion that there might be something physically responsible for preventing a pregnancy to occur.

That same month, a friend told me about something I had never considered before—acupuncture. Acupuncture, you say? You mean that pin-cushion-Hellraiser-looking Eastern medicine, voodoo guru-type stuff where they poke, prod, and brainwash you into a state of total relaxation and then take all your money and spend it on Tiki god worship? Ummm . . . yes. No! Well, I mean to say I had my reservations about it all.

I had just spent all my effort, time, and prayers entering into a place of peace with my very own Jesus, and here I was considering a practice some might consider questionable in its origin, success, and legitimacy. Yes, I did my homework. I didn't take any new course of action lightly, and I wasn't about to hand over the reins of my peace to someone holding a stack of needles without a good reason.

This is not an ad for acupuncture. I'm not here to convince you that it will fix all your ailments or cure you of the common cold, let alone infertility. What I will tell you is that it is not voodoo and it is not scary. My very-experienced doctor was friendly and thorough, answered all my questions, and encouraged me that if no baby came of these efforts, I would be left with a more relaxed body at the very least. That sounded safe and splendid to me, so . . . I had fertility acupuncture.

The month I had acupuncture was a weird month for us. Josh had a business trip that took him out of town for a few days, and I flew home to Kansas for a while after that to spend some time with my dad who was recovering from knee surgery. Needless to say, we were very nearly two proverbial baby-making ships passing in the night, so our realistic hopes were not high for this to be the month of our long-awaited conception of a child.

Upon my return from Kansas, I was struck with an unexplained urinary tract infection followed by unimaginable back pain. I had experienced brutal back pain before in my life. I even passed out from a pinched sciatic nerve a few years prior, and the feeling of waking up in an ER with a morphine drip was not an experience I was longing to relive any time soon. Valentine's night, instead of going out to a romantic dinner reminiscing about memories of our undying love for each other, I found myself agonizing in pain at the doctor's office. I spent the night on the couch, hopped up on painkillers and attempting to make the most of what was left of our night of romance by not spilling too many black beans from my Chipotle burrito on myself as I ate in a Roman-style lounge-while-eating position. You know you married well when your husband can still look at you and smile as you numbly gnaw on a burrito in the horizontal position. Yep, he's a keeper.

The next week was filled with more doctor appointments. I took a pregnancy test each morning "just in case," followed by a frown of disappointment followed by another round of heavy painkillers to help me hobble through another day on the couch. To cap off that weekend, I woke up Monday morning to my period. I was in too much pain to be surprised and was in all honesty slightly relieved to know that all the painkillers I had been taking were okay since I was, in fact, not pregnant again. I was on enough medication that I was unable to drive myself, so Josh took me to my appointment to get an X-ray that next day.

"Any chance you are pregnant?" the radiologist asked me as I lay on the table while she positioned the lead plates and X-ray tube to target my source of pain.

"No," I said. "We are trying, but I just got my period today and I tested negative this morning, just in case."

The X-ray showed nothing. Another round of painkillers and another lecture on taking it easy and I was sent home again.

The next day my pain continued, but my period disappeared. Two days of negative tests later, I found my pain had doubled. It wasn't just in my back, but now my entire middle was consumed by a cramping so severe I felt like I was being crushed by an inner tube of inexplicable torture. I took my prescribed medication and went to bed.

The next morning I woke up pregnant.

You think *you're* shocked by the news? Ten months, two weeks, six days, and four hours into our journey of conception, and I find myself standing like a hunchback in our bathroom in the wee hours of the morning staring blurry-eyed at a measly testing strip from the local Dollar Tree. My pee had just turned it from bright white into one stripe of pink and one stripe of definitely *not* nothing there as reality started to creep into my brain with the utmost of horror and shock. *What*?!

Needless to say, four dipsticks and one digital test blinking PREGNANT later, I found myself hyperventilating in a scene that was a very far cry from the ecstatic moment of joy I had pictured in my head for so long. First things first. I woke up Josh with a scream of happiness from the bathroom. His disturbed sleep cycle instantaneously turned from perturbed to elated as we found ourselves jumping for joy (well, he was jumping. I was doing more of a dysfunctional shrug-type motion, but still!) in our tiny bathroom.

Surreal joy was quickly mixed with acute fear at the obvious questions we had surrounding my current state of pain. We called my parents. We called my doctor. Within hours, I found myself feet-up, holding my husband's hand, staring at an ultrasound screenshot of our baby. Our. Baby.

The entire world melted away. All the pain and meds and anxieties and fears and questions and impossibilities of the universe disappeared for a split second as my mind got lost somewhere between my heart and that black-and-white, grainy, five-inch screen that proved beyond a reasonable doubt that inside my body, right at that moment, a new human being was forming.

Outside of reason. Outside of percentages and chances and bets. Outside of my control, my planning, my actions or my wildest dreams.

I was looking at my child.

9

Flutters and Butterflies

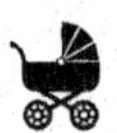

I was expecting when I least expected it. The fears of that first day finding out we were pregnant were only a glimmer of the emotions we were about to experience. After a week of bed rest and much prayer my back pain was all but gone, only to be explained by the unusual amount of stretching and cramping a new baby caused by turning my uterus into a home for the next nine months. The X-rays and painkillers had no effect on the baby, and I was relieved to see the look of confidence on the faces of my doctors as they reassured me that all was well. Still, the joy I felt in knowing I was carrying new life was the best medicine I could have received, and two weeks later I was back to my usual self, back on my feet, and back at work (back puns intended.)

We let our immediate family know we were expecting right away. We wanted as many prayers as possible with such a tumultuous start out of the gate. Oh, and remember that fertility appointment I had put on the calendar just a couple months prior? With a beaming smile, I ended up making the call and changing that appointment into my first prenatal visit! (Good work, God, reminding me how I am sincerely on Your calendar after all!)

IS THAT BLOB ON THE SCREEN MY BABY?

The day of my first prenatal appointment, I was suspected to be about seven weeks along. This was going to be our first ultrasound since that scary trip to the ER, and we woke up excited and nervous, not exactly knowing what was in store. I had been feeling pretty good, just a couple days into a wee bit of nausea, but nothing more. The appointment was in the afternoon, so we both had to work all morning as if it was just a usual day. Since we worked at the same university, it was nice to know there was at least one other person nearby who knew my current state, but for the most part I felt like an undercover agent.

A few hours into the morning, I made a casual trip to the rest room and I found some spotting. My heart skipped a beat. I tried not to panic. Was it just nerves? Was I going to miscarry? What's wrong? I texted Josh and then called the doctor immediately. Since we were already planning to see the doctor within a few hours, all I could do was wait. Wait! Needless to say, that did not help my level of distraction sitting at work for the next few hours. I think I must have made about seventeen trips to the bathroom that morning. I wanted to leave. I wanted to rest. I wanted answers, and I wanted them immediately. I doubt anyone ever prayed so much in that little bathroom stall than I did that morning. I was scared out of my mind.

I met Josh in the main lobby, and we held hands as we walked to the car. I don't think I had ever held his hand so nervously since the day of our wedding, and just like on that day, with the touch of his hand I knew we were going to make it. We prayed, we took a deep breath, and we drove the long drive to the doctor (well, really it was only about seven miles, but it might as well have been seven light years away in that moment.)

We met our OB/GYN and were thankful for her kindness and reassuring smile as she rolled out the little in-office ultrasound machine. I felt so blessed to live in a place and time where there even existed equipment such as the ultrasound. I have no idea how these machines really work or who invented them or even how long they have really been around, but I would absolutely kiss whoever was that first person to say "let's figure out a way to see the baby *before* it is born." Bravo, person, thank you!

The doctor maneuvered the device until she found a good picture (and by good I mean the grainy blizzard of specks on the screen could be deciphered by her eyes only.) Her face was stoic but relaxed. I tried to read her emotions for any hint of relief, but she just studied the images silently as we waited with baited breath.

"See that flutter?" She finally spoke.

We both squinted at the screen. It looked like a weird maze inside a black balloon. You could have told me I was looking at the image of a distant unknown galaxy in outer space and I would have totally believed you. And then, as if I was glaring at one of those silly, trick computer images with the invisible image hidden in the print (you know, from the 1990s that your aunt and uncle had framed in their bathroom that looked like a gritty rainbow until you stared at it so long it changed into a giant pirate ship with seagulls flying overhead? Right.) I could suddenly make sense of what I was seeing. A flutter. A quick blink of black and white that was steady and fast and altogether unworldly.

"That's the baby's heartbeat," the doctor said. She spoke it so suddenly that my mind couldn't keep up with my emotions. I was crying with joy before my brain could even comprehend the reality. We were on top of the roller coaster once more, catching our breath from the knowledge that once again everything was just fine. Unbelievable. We were only seven weeks into this pregnancy, and the ebb and flow of worry and bliss felt nearly unbearable. And yet, all I wanted was more. I don't mean to say I wanted more to worry about. The thought that something could truly be wrong with our baby was unfathomable, but the level of happiness, love, and gratitude that came with each ounce of good news we received was more wondrous than I ever could have expected. I was starting to understand that this cycle of concern and gratitude was going to be part of a permanent cast of feelings transforming us into parents.

And, oh yeah, we were becoming parents and nobody knew it yet! Well, besides our close family, anyway. But now, armed with a black-and-white photo from the ultrasound, we had the proof to show for it. It's a hard decision to make as to when to break the news. I had read up on different stories about cute ways to make the big announcement, and really I just wanted to hire a skywriter and shout it from the rooftops!

There is also the "friend politics" to consider. Oh c'mon, you know what I mean. "If So and So hears it from someone else besides us . . ." or "Don't post anything on Facebook before we tell So and So" and so forth. It is so tricky these days to prioritize how to roll out major news. You don't want anyone to feel left out because they didn't hear it from you personally. You also want to be there to actually confirm the news so that any questions of rumor are dismissed before they begin. (Has she just been eating too many donuts or is she pregnant?) But we were so bursting at the seams to share our excitement that in less than twenty-four hours after that first appointment the entire world (well, world who knew us, anyway) learned of our joy. *THE PARDYS ARE HAVING A BABY* might as well have been tattooed on my forehead. Somehow just after officially announcing it at work, updating my Facebook status, and tweeting the news, I think I managed to start just about every conversation with some reference to my new condition. I couldn't help myself. Maybe it was the hormones, maybe it was the relief of finally saying it out loud, maybe it was just the increased gravitational pull around my slowly-growing-to-the-size-of-a-planet belly, but I wanted the world to revolve around me and my happiness that day.

MIRACLES, MIGRAINES, AND MORNING SICKNESS

It was like living in a dream. Some mornings I'd wake up reminding myself that, even though I couldn't see it or feel it, there was a *child* growing inside my own body. A new human. An entirely unknown being no one had ever met before. A creation that was completely unique and individual and already loved beyond words.

Other mornings were not so pleasant. All that stuff you hear about the first trimester being wrought with pangs of joy and misery—well, it's pretty much true. You are as happy as you are nauseous, which is a lot and often, for the most part. What I lacked in vomit I made up for in migraines. No lie—I had a horrible headache for fourteen weeks straight. Yes, it sucked. Yes, there were times I wanted to nap at work. Yes, I pretty much wanted to punch my unsympathetic, nonpregnant, male coworkers in the face every day. Yes, as thrilled as I was to have brought this on myself and to have prayed fervently for months to be in this condition, it felt like it was entirely unreasonable and unfair to live day in and day out in an exhausted state of ugh-i-ness.

I wanted to whine and moan and have someone offer to give me piggyback rides so I didn't have to walk anywhere anymore. I wanted my boss to tell me I could just magically take the next month off and only do tasks I felt like doing (nothing.) I wanted those stupid B vitamins and anti-nausea lozenges and Mommy-to-be teas to work their magic and actually do what they promised on the box and make me feel as happy and energetic as the smiling pregnant woman advertised on the front of the package. I just wanted to feel good—the end.

And just when I thought I couldn't take it anymore, week fifteen brought relief, comfort, and Coca-Cola. Yes, it's true. I had been caffeine-free ever since I had started trying to conceive. I was really, truly trying to be good about what I put into my body, how I fed it and treated it and took care of it. But you try having a freaking vice around your brain for fourteen weeks straight and then judge me after one bottle of Coca-Cola brought me the first moment of relief I had felt in months. Aww, sweet satisfaction.

10

Count Your Blessings and Your Calories

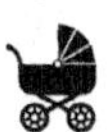

Here is the thing about pregnancy that I learned in the first trimester: Every pregnancy for each woman is entirely different. You might have ideals in your head of how you think you will be/react/respond to your body growing a new human. You might have thoughts or plans or extremely specific demands when it comes to considering how you will adapt to this new state of feeling. I know it seems perfect and lovely and even right to think about only eating organically, counting every ounce of protein, waking up and smiling through prenatal yoga positions, maintaining your correct posture, and keeping your body active. Just throw that in the trash. Seriously. Just kill that dream right here and now. Look, I'm not saying there won't be those days. I'm not saying it's impossible. But, really, I am. It is. It's impossible. That's not what pregnancy looks like, especially in the first trimester. And sure, it was hard for me to sip that Coke and look my stringently-organic friends in the eyes some days. But you know what? I was actually doing what was best for me, and that stupid soda made me feel fantastic.

Obviously, you're going to do the best you can. You

should read the books, certainly stop drinking alcohol or (heaven forbid) smoking (no, seriously, stop) and work to eat healthier and be healthier than you've ever been in your entire life. You have the greatest motivating factor growing inside your body right now that will help propel you away from the Twinkies and directly to the produce aisle, no doubt. But listen to your body and your doctor, not your friends. No one else is carrying this baby every day. No one else is craving that cheeseburger at three in the morning that you know is the only thing that will suppress your nausea. No one else is going to drag your listless body through yet another workday and see to it that you are resting enough for two people.

Take care of yourself and don't be stupid. But, by golly, if all that is standing between your grimacing discomfort and a valley of relief is a measly bottle of Coca-cola (or a cheeseburger or a bag of M&Ms or a carton of Ben & Jerry's) then don't let other people's notions of idealism guilt you out of that. Drink the Coke. Feel better. Move on. Moderation, not guilt, will get you much further down the road towards the pregnancy of your dreams.

The second trimester was a breeze, so to speak. They always say it will be your best, and it truly is. You have the cute belly to prove to the world of passersby that you are, indeed and without a doubt, "in the family way." Yet you have not quite grown to blimp-o-rama status where everyone cringes in pity when they glance your way. No, no, this is the joyous time when you actually feel pretty good about your body, your growing baby, and you might not even mind the occasional tummy pat from the strange, elderly woman you are stuck with on the elevator that day.

But, boy oh boy, is that body a-changin'! I always wondered, of course, what it would be like to be pregnant. I remember trying to conjure up the idea of something moving inside me or carrying extra pounds that were not just a sore reflection of a giant burrito I couldn't put down the night before. So here I was, packing on the mommy tummy and finally feeling my baby start to kick for the first time, and the only way I could describe it to my inquisitive husband was this: It feels exactly how you think it would feel. Brilliant, I know. But entirely true. And weird. We can't forget weird.

The changes pregnancy brings to your body are literally indescribable. It is sort of crazy to me that there are even books on it at all, because as much as we want to know what is normal or okay or what might actually be signs for alarm, it seems nearly impossible to describe on paper how you are actually going to be feeling from the inside out. Medical progress aside, there is nothing in the books that tells you anything about the fact that every time your husband puts his hand on your belly the baby will stop kicking at that exact same moment. There is nothing to be found about how giddy you will get just sitting at your cubicle in the middle of the workday counting the tiny jolts your belly makes each time your baby hiccups. And you won't find anything out there that can tell you why in the world it feels good to have your baby head-butt your bladder simply because the sensation allows you yet another moment to be amazed at the miracle inside you. Pregnancy is as close to real-life, fairy-tale magic as our bodies will ever come.

But as you know, in every fairy tale there is always a villain. (No, don't worry, I'm not referring to the baby!) The villain in this story is known as Body Image, and this is just the beginning (we'll see more of him post-baby.)

TOO MANY DONUTS OR A BABY BUMP?

I always hated my stomach. Hated it. Thanks to my lucky gene pool, that particular area became my trouble spot early in my teens, and I can still remember the first time someone asked me if I was pregnant when I wasn't. (I was only seventeen and wearing a bathing suit with a skirt—double ouch!) By my early twenties, I had a new reason to hate my stomach—my high levels of anxiety had led me to develop rather severe IBS (irritable bowel syndrome) and I was plagued with horrible cramps that seemed relentless no matter the measures I took. I was uncomfortable. I was sad. I was completely disillusioned with the idea that "if only" my stomach were flat and beautiful I could finally get on with living a lovely and definitely not-looking-pregnant-when-I-wasn't lifestyle.

By the time I was newly married in my mid-to-late twenties, I had come a long way. A painful path and an enormous dose of perspective had helped me call a truce with my midsection. That isn't to say I exchanged my Spanx for crop tops! Heavens, no. But growing up has a funny way of showing you that the people who really love and support you are not sticking by your side due to what you look like. Period. Above all, I'd married a man who simply wouldn't stand for the fact that I wanted to speak lies about myself as if they were fact. I was no longer allowed to put myself down, and that was that. It was the healthiest habit I've ever formed in my life—replacing insults with gratitude. (It's much harder than it sounds!)

So it's ironic to imagine a former belly-hater eager to get pregnant and get growing, but I was. Maybe it was the fact that it had taken so long to conceive. Maybe it was the fact that every little movement inside me now perplexed me to my core. Or maybe it was, at least a little, the fact that for the next nine-ish months I didn't have to worry about sucking it in or pretending I wasn't pregnant—I was!

I'll admit I never minded people thinking I was pregnant when I actually was even at ten weeks when my belly was barely popping and I was definitely still in the donuts-or-baby questionable zone of development. But there was more to my newfound belly appreciation than just the fashionable tent dresses I was now allowed to comfortably sport.

BUMP LOVE

For the first time in my life, I loved my belly. LOVED. Here it was, full of baby and beautifully bulging. Sure, I was gaining discomfort by the minute. Yes, I protruded so earnestly that I had to wear one of those ugly support belts to help me not topple over and strain my back. Absolutely, I had the worst gas of my entire life that seemed less and less controllable with each passing day. But my belly was housing my child, plain and simple.

My belly had finally become my ally. It was functioning properly and perfectly, and God knew what He was doing when he tucked it right in our middle, stationed right between our arms and able to be hugged at all times. I knew there would come a time when this baby would be outside of my body, even beyond the reach of my hands, but right now the only thing that mattered was how my body was not failing me at all. It was providing enormous protection and keeping my sweet child safe. And, frankly, I really had nothing to do with it! God is amazing how He designed the pregnant woman to function on autopilot while every tiny cell and molecule and atom lines up perfectly in place and finds its path to developing life.

My belly had become the epicenter of *remarkable*. Nothing could ever take that away from me. And feeling this child wriggle and squirm in me became a constant reminder that my belly wasn't the only thing expanding. My concepts of love and gratitude were bursting at the seams as well. To take a step back, to even consider dislike towards my body after experiencing something so incredible—that would be like smacking God Himself in the face. How could I feel anything but love for something that was clearly a living, breathing blessing in my life? My body was a walking miracle housing another miracle. And now you see why maybe it is impossible to describe how that feels from the inside out!

11

When Blue or Pink Isn't So Black and White

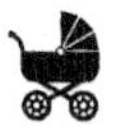

Just as I was starting to get used to the idea that a little human was inside me, I began relentlessly wondering exactly *who* it was in there. I'll cut to the chase—was it a boy or a girl? Every person I know seems to have their own opinion as to why or why not you should or should not find out the gender of the baby. Certainly, this is for each couple to decide for themselves. I'll explain my own motivations.

I'd heard it all:

"You will never get a bigger surprise than that in your entire life."

"There is nothing like that feeling of finding out on their birthday."

"It helped motivate me to want to push harder and find out!"

And so on and so forth.

But no matter what, nothing was going to stop me from finding out as soon as possible if we were about to shop for pink or blue. My reason? I figured there is enough surprise that comes with a baby already. There is an entire universe full of mysteries and unsolvable answers and questions greater than I can even fathom, so I say let's remove as much ambiguity as possible in the beginning so I can have the mental energy to focus on what is unknown once that baby does arrive. Besides, it is going to be a surprise either way, and I'd rather not be screaming in agony when I get to realize whether I'm having a son or a daughter.

About halfway through the pregnancy they do what's called an anatomy ultrasound where they not only can check the gender of the baby but also make sure the tiny body is developing properly.

My husband and I took the whole day off work. Again, we found it a good time to pause, celebrate, and savor the moment that our lives were about to change. I imagined what our family photos would look like. Would there be a little girl in tutus and bows or father and son in matching argyle sweater vests? (Ha!)

The night before the ultrasound I could hardly sleep. To be honest, for the whole week or two leading up to that night I found myself restless with excitement. For years I had dreamt about this child, and since the day we heard the heartbeat this was my first real step in getting to know who my child was.

Certainly, we "didn't care" what sex the baby would be. I mean, that's what you are supposed to say anyway, right? Everyone just wants a healthy baby. The luxury of the firstborn child is that it really doesn't seem to matter if it is a girl or boy since, in our case anyway, we didn't plan on having an only child. This was just *numero uno* for us. So it wasn't so much about wanting this or that, but of course we had our inclinations.

Josh thought it was a girl, absolutely. I admit I was sort of hopeful for a girl, but both my brother and sister had boys as their firstborns, so I knew it may be a good chance there was a boy in there. I really wasn't sure. We talked about girl names and boy names and what the nursery theme might be and so forth. The first trimester allows for the most dreaming since you really can't get down to hammering out the details until you know more (or at least until you feel up to it!)

So there I was, lying in bed the night before the big day, dreaming of my baby boy or girl. I couldn't wrap my brain around the idea that right there, right then, I didn't know. It was unknown. I lay still, soaking up this feeling of utter possibility and tried to imagine the moment of going from unknowing to knowing in a single second. I imagined the ultrasound tech saying the words *it's a boy/girl* and attempted to guess what emotions I'd have in hearing such news. It was weird. It was this out-of-body mind game to envision myself and all my thoughts, ideas, hopes, and possible futures transferring from one place—the unknown—to the solidified, actual reality of knowing what was to come. That's about as good as I can explain it.

In the waiting room of the radiology department, I rubbed my round belly in anticipation of the news. No matter what amazingly happy news of his or her gender was to come, there was going to be a loss of one dream no matter what. I was so excited to find out if the baby was a boy or girl that I barely had the capacity to expect any kind of disappointment at all. After all, this was our first baby. I simply and wholly and completely just wanted good and healthy news. So that is where I directed my prayers, certainly. Besides, the gender was already decided whether I knew it or not. My knowing wouldn't change the fact of who was in there.

Forty-five minutes of a gelled-up, globby belly later, the tech was ready to call Josh back into the ultrasound room so we could have a clear look-see at who was inside there. We held our breath, squinted at the screen, and tried our best to decipher baby parts in the black-and-white nonsensical blizzard on the monitor.

She was a girl! And she was perfectly healthy.

A girl! We were beaming. We were crying. We were staring at our *daughter*, and it felt like my heart swelled up straight into my throat as I comprehended the pink and precocious possibilities of our determined future. A GIRL. We could not have felt more gratitude, happiness, or love in a single moment.

We made the phone calls. We posted the Facebook news and were elated to share the fact that a Pardy girl was on her way. As we got back in the car and took a deep breath of sheer joy, it took me a minute to discover a strange but tiny void.

It's a strange sensation. It's not exactly a loss. As they say, how can you lose something you never had? But I had to take a minute to grieve the loss of the possibility of having a first-born son. It's not that I would have preferred a son. It's not that I even thought I was going to have a son. But just as I would have grieved the potential of having a daughter if it was the other way around, I had to stop and intentionally adjust my habit of dreaming about various possibilities.

I was in the know now. I was having a daughter. A daughter! Ah, and the gratitude and joy I held for that new knowledge quickly swelled into the place of the new void, expanding itself into my whole being, and the grief I felt for losing the dream of unknowing was replaced forever. It was only a moment of acknowledgement, of sadness, of lament, but it was an important step for me in being able to completely move on and entirely embrace the truth and truly enjoy the newfound knowledge of my daughter's pending arrival.

My daughter. I couldn't get over it! I hugged my belly and closed my eyes and started picturing this darling, this beauty, this sweet, pink baby who would be all mine to love and spoil forever.

This wiggly little bundle of belly was also a constant reminder that a clock was ticking. A clock that was telling me to get ready, prep for, and welcome an actual new human into our very own not-so-child-friendly abode.

12

Growing to the Size of a Small Planet "Just for the Fun of It"

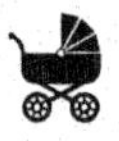

Armed with this newly-pink and precious baby knowledge, we found ourselves thrown into the lion's den of baby preparation. That is, Babies R Us.

If there ever were a place where the happiness of welcoming a baby goes to die it would be Babies R Us. Okay, okay, I kid (mostly.) It starts off as a pleasant shopping trip full of wonder and excitement, and three exhausting hours later when you've scanned all the merchandise you aren't even sure is essential to child rearing, the trip has turned into a necessary evil you wouldn't wish on your worst enemy.

NAVIGATING A FOREIGN COUNTRY (OR REGISTERING FOR BABY STUFF)

Registering for baby stuff is brutal. Brace yourself. Pace yourself. And face the fact that there is absolutely no getting around it. You have to do it. Even if you have a billion dollars and no friends and are planning on buying everything for yourselves—in which case, maybe you should put down this book and head straight to therapy and then call me up for coffee so we can chat about being friends and you sharing your wealth with me—there will no doubt still be *someone* who finds out you are having a baby and wants to send you something and wants to see what you need and wants to know what brand or theme or color you have chosen for the wee one.

You might be thinking, "Registering sounds great! I want to do it! I'm looking forward to it!" And you should think that. You should because we all do, and if we didn't think that way we would never walk through the sliding doors of baby merchandise wonderland.

But remember back when you were engaged? Remember how much you *loved* your fiancé and it sounded soooo exciting to register together? It would be a nice break away from wedding planning to stop chattering about which centerpieces or appetizers to have at the reception and go pick out things that other people can buy for you and your new love shack. It started off all nice and sweet, and you liked picking out tablecloths while he enjoyed shooting things with the scan gun. You were having a great time until two hours into it he rolled his eyes at you when you couldn't decide between the brown towels or the tan towels, and pretty soon it escalated into a full-on debate over whether one should have six or eight salad plates and you were glaring at each other with laser-beam eyes in the middle of Target and you were pretty sure the employees circling you had a pool going on who would be the first to break the staring match. (Congratulations on winning—was it worth it?)

So imagine something like that. But instead of tablecloths and towels it is mountains of strollers and aisles of breast pumps, all of which look impossible to distinguish from one another and none of which you know how to operate or put together. It's sort of like landing in a foreign country and totally nodding, acting like you know what everyone else is saying, even though it feels like everything they are saying is a joke about you and how you don't know what you're doing.

You are going to feel lost, and that's okay. Before you go, ask a friend who is already a mom to walk you through her house, if you can. Just see what she has. Ask her what she bought and never used. Ask her why she chose the brands she did. Ask her what broke three days after she got it. Ask her what not to buy. Take a few notes, evaluate the size of the space you have to prepare, and read a few reviews online about some of the essentials. Safety and convenience should be at the top of your priority list, not cuteness and snuggly-ness. The baby will bring enough of that. You really don't need to register for it.

People are going to be more generous than you expect. Your friends will help you more than you think. And your baby will not starve (even if you try out the breast pump on your cat before yourself) or go cold (even if you don't buy that insanely-soft, plush blanket that costs more than your wedding dress) or care which car seat you put them in (even if it is brown and not pink and someone will say what a lovely son you have every time you place her in it.)

QUEEN FOR A DAY

The day of my baby shower I felt like a queen. A very enormous, waddling queen. Like one of those dancing ballerina hippos in the sequence from *Fantasia* that always seemed very trippy but sweet. I didn't know what to expect, really. I had five very generous friends offer to throw me a shower at one of their houses, and I told them I just wanted to feel pretty and eat cake basically, so as long as there was something there with frosting on it I was going to be a happy gal. My mom came out for the occasion, and we got pedicures before heading to my friend's house.

Now I have to sidestep for a second and bring you up to speed on how my actual pregnancy was coming along, because I don't want you to miss out on one very important fact here—I was huge. No, no, don't get me wrong. I was supposed to be growing. I was, after all, supporting a human life inside my own body. When I looked in the mirror I liked what I saw, a glowing (albeit sweaty) face and an expanding belly nourishing life inside. I felt beautiful. But I was enormous.

At work there were particular people who could not help but comment every single time they spotted me. One woman who worked in a neighboring department would walk out of her way just to tell me how insanely big I looked. No lie. I tried to avoid eye contact with her. I even found myself staying in the stall of the women's rest room a few minutes longer to prevent interaction with her if I noticed she was in there at the same time. It was ridiculous. This may sound extreme, but after someone stops you for the fifth day in a row to say "Are you very sure you aren't having twins?" you just try to bypass them altogether.

It was true that I was bigger than the average pregnant lady. My doctor would measure my fundus (I always hated that term—it sounded like a rotting foot disease to me.) That is the length of the belly in centimeters from the top of the uterus to the bottom, and my doctor let me know that at most appointments I was measuring ahead of schedule. It wasn't unhealthy or anything to be worried about, just big. It didn't help matters that I am naturally short-torsoed. My baby simply had nowhere to go but outward! So I carried my beach-ball belly proudly. What else was I to do? If people wanted to ogle me, by all means take a picture. It would last longer.

Now on this particular day of my party, as my mother and I were getting prettied and pedicured and treating ourselves to a moment of beauty, I was feeling great sitting there and trusting that the sweet lady at my feet was doing a good job, since I actually couldn't see my toes, when I looked over and noticed another pregnant lady next to me.

Being pregnant and running into other pregnant ladies is a phenomenon all its own. You can't help but compare belly shapes and sizes. You guess due dates and genders, and in a split second you size up what kind of mother you think she will be. It's awkward and unwarranted but entirely true. You always leave the encounter thinking you're the winner (or you should anyway) and that your baby will certainly come out cuter and more loved than hers ever could. This might sound sick, but I think it is something innate in those crazy pregnancy hormones that enables you to build up the amount of protective mama-bear strength you are going to need later when you're gearing up to push a watermelon out of your bum (so to speak.)

This other pregnant lady and her mother were also having a day of beauty (go figure) so we swapped baby facts about ourselves. Sure enough, this lady was just a few weeks ahead of me and about half my size. I gripped the arms of the massage chair and literally bit my tongue in anticipation of the avalanche of gawking that was about to pour down on me. Sure enough.

Her mother audibly gasped. I'll never forget it. My mother tried to come to my defense, offering sweet compliments like how I "carry just like she did" and so on. But it was no use. The mother-daughter duo just kept at it. They simply could not comprehend the fact that I was so enormous carrying only one baby and as far along as I was.

Just when I'd had enough, when I was debating whether I should fake labor or punch her in the face, I looked down at my sweet belly and remembered how much I loved it. Okay, maybe I still wanted to punch them both in the face (those hormones aren't diffused so easily with one belly glance) but I just smiled and exclaimed proudly, "I know! I'm a walking marvel!" The end.

Nothing was going to steal my moment in the sun for me. They could try all they wanted. They might even eclipse the sun for moment, interrupting the natural light. But, as science would have it, when the sun is eclipsed the light shines even brighter, more intensely, and all the more beautifully than it did before. Bring it on, you silly women! You're only going to reveal to me how much more miraculous and impossibly marvelous my daughter is! It *is* amazing that my body can stretch as far as it can! It *is* incredible that my organs are still functioning when they are being squeezed so entirely out of the way by my gigantic baby. It *is* unbelievable that I can still go to work and sit up by myself and carry on with a smile on my face when I'm carrying such a load. Because pregnancy is sheer awesomeness wrapped in overwhelming joy dipped in breathtaking wonder and candy-coated in remarkable, amazing, humbling, astounding splendor! How's that for a reminder?

My baby shower was amazing. In the days before Pinterest

and trying to one-up each other on how customized you can make everything these days, you would have thought by the looks of my shower that my friends invented those ideas. I felt special, loved, and . . . awkward.

Okay, so here is the truth about baby showers. You sort of imagine something like a birthday party yet more reception-like but centered around you and your baby, a time when you get to celebrate something none of you really know anything about—your baby—who hasn't even arrived yet. And that's the weird part. You open the gifts, you tell the stories, you cut the cake, and suddenly you realize that maybe for the first time ever in your life you are celebrating someone else's life. It's like going to someone else's birthday party and opening their presents for them when they don't show up.

I don't mean to sound ungrateful. On the contrary, I was speechless with thanks. But as I unwrapped sweet baby girl onesies and opened bags of quilts and diapers and teething rings, I felt this overwhelming sensation that I was thankful not just *for* this baby but *on behalf* of her. She was her own person, with needs and thoughts and emotions, and now a closet full of clothes and blankies and toys!

There was another speechless, heart-stopping moment at my shower I would be remiss not to mention. I don't know where he got the idea, but I hope each of you reading this steal it and make it your own whenever you can. My husband, without me knowing, recorded himself speaking to the baby and me and telling us how much he loved us. Since it was just a for-women-only kind of shower, it gave him the opportunity to "be" there and be part of the whole experience while also taking time to thank me for my ever-expanding wonder belly and to state how incredibly excited and nervous and happy he was in anticipation of our daughter. It is a moment I will never forget (and don't have to, since I have the DVD to watch and rewatch whenever I like) and it had all us gals teary with romance by the end of it. A video, a letter, or some kind of sentiment from the daddy-to-be (even if done in private) is something he will never regret taking time to do.

My baby shower had come and gone. The nursery was

painted (painstakingly striped every two inches by my husband in two shades of pink and yellow.) The closet was full (0-3 months washed, older clothes hanging according to size and season.) The house was clean (even the baseboards were scrubbed) and our arms were open and ready. And so we waited.

13

Goldilocks and the Three Birth Plans

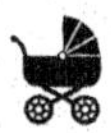

In the weeks leading up to "go time" we found ourselves restlessly reviewing our plan of action. That is, our birth plan.

In the second trimester we talked with our doctor about what options awaited us for labor and delivery. I read and read and read all the birth stories online I could stomach and came to the conclusion that if it was possible to endure a natural birth I would certainly be up for attempting it. It seemed to me it was at least worth a try, and if drugs or intervention could be avoided then I should educate myself as much as possible on what I could expect. I researched various natural birthing methods and found The Bradley Method to be a good fit for us.

HIPPIES OR HOSPITALS?

The thing is, there seems to be two camps when it comes to choosing a birth plan. I never liked this, as stereotyping never reflects well on anyone. On one hand, you have the big, bad doctors who form a giant, numbers-driven conglomerate out to surgically remove your baby in an assembly line of selfish, pharmaceutically-financed, brainwashed, money-mongering, medical robots who don't care about you or your level of comfort and convenience. On the other, you have the flowery hippies who live on flaxseed oil and organic raw foods and practice hours of stretching and meditation and see no reason you can't catch your own baby with your own bare hands with a smile on your face and amniotic fluid on your bedroom floor and welcome your new baby (no doubt named something like Harvest or Storm or Tulip or Pumpkin) with chants of starry verses made up from whatever song you are feeling in your heart at the moment.

Choose your camp wisely.

I couldn't bring myself to do it. I refused to wholly enter in to either of these scenarios and never found comfort placing my trust (let alone my uterus) in the hands of one or the other. I became adamant about discovering a hybrid that suited my needs.

If there was ever a time to become your own health advocate—and surround yourself with a few good supporters—pregnancy is it. I wanted and needed (based on some of my own medical history) to have the birth in the hospital. I wanted the experience to be happy and calm. I wanted to be asked and told what was going on at all times. I wanted Josh to be equally educated on what my body was up to. I wanted to feel secure in my answers when I was asked what I wanted in the midst of labor. I wanted to leave the hospital with a healthy baby that was my own, and anything else beyond that was negotiable, bottom line.

We found and took part in a local twelve-week Bradley Method class. It offered advice, information, and simple education on relaxation methods and labor progression. It gave Josh the confidence he needed to feel like he was actively participating in the birth just as much as I was (well, nearly anyway . . . let's be realistic here.)

No doubt, we are forever grateful for this education. It didn't leave me feeling like I knew more than the doctors. (I don't, and unless you are an OB neither do you.) But I did understand my body, my baby, and my preferences for nearly all potential scenarios that awaited us. For me, knowledge was power and power was peace when it came to anticipating the unknown. I didn't know how it would all roll out, but I did know what to do (for the most part) when it happened, and that brought much relief to my nerves.

You might not find your perfect birth plan in a book. You might not read about it online or hear of it from any of your friends. You might have to completely make it up on your own and customize your own priorities and ask for things you deem valuable, because your doctor or your mother or your husband might not have any idea otherwise. And by the time you need something or recognize your desires, it might be too late to make them happen for you. So if you aren't going to take a birthing class (which I sincerely hope you do) or write out an actual birth plan (also encouraged) then at least have a conversation with those closest to you about what you hope for, expect, and need when you are at your worst. Because, trust me, when contractions get going things get real ugly real quick, and nobody can read your mind even if you are screaming at them to shut up and get you your ChapStick.

IT'S ALL FUN AND GAMES UNTIL SOMEONE'S WATER BREAKS

We spent the nights leading up to my due date in the nursery, dreaming. I rocked in the glider and Josh usually sprawled himself out in the middle of the floor, stretching and taking deep sighs as we vocalized our impatience on awaiting this child. We would take walks, eat spicy food, and try just about anything to turn these darn Braxton Hicks contractions into real and actual contractions. To no avail. Nevertheless, the time was coming, and we knew I couldn't be pregnant forever, right?

Looking back and remembering is one thing. I could tell you that you won't forget certain feelings or pains or thoughts you have when you actually give birth. But the truth is, some thoughts and feelings are lost very quickly after you get that baby in your arms. This is one reason I recorded my birth story almost immediately following her birth. I didn't want to forget. Here you have it—the actual (and not too gruesome, for those of you still in the first trimester with weak stomachs) account of the birth of my first daughter, written just days after she arrived:

> It was Halloween night (cue eerie music now) and we had just been over at a friend's house. They have a little girl, so we all took her trick-or-treating, hoping that the walk would do me some good (and hopefully spur on labor.) Many people had questioned whether I was hiding a giant pumpkin under my shirt or not. Jokes were made like "It's the Great Pumpkin, Charlie Brown" and with good reason—I was downright enormous. I had walked miles that week trying to induce contractions but to no avail.
>
> We went home, having eaten spicy chili and way too much Halloween candy. We started to watch "Dracula" on TV, and I mentioned to Josh that I was determined to "scare this baby out of me!"
>
> I was technically due November third, but people had been commenting for weeks that I looked overdue, even my own doctors. I still believe I was a couple of weeks past due, though I was truly thankful for every minute of pregnancy. I had a fairly uneventful pregnancy and enjoyed every little movement, little kick, little amazing hiccup that Matilda made in the womb. In fact (and this is not romanticized—you can ask my husband) I worried that I would miss her once she was delivered. I am one of those crazy ladies that most other pregnant women hate—the one wearing the smile right up until the end. But, in God's perfect timing, I did finally feel ready to actually meet her that week. I had recently had extra swelling and itchiness all over my body that was signaling to me this pregnancy needed to come to a close and it wouldn't be long before she would be out.
>
> So we were watching "Dracula" at home (thankfully) and at 10 p.m. exactly I was laying on the couch watching the movie when I heard a pop and felt something like a kick in the pelvic bone from the inside. I was like "Whoa" and ran to the bathroom 'cause I knew it was unlike anything I had ever felt before. It was seriously just like out of the movies

(even though they warn you "it will be nothing like it is in the movies" ha ha.)

I yelled from the bathroom, "I think my water broke!" I was shocked and instantly felt giddy and excited and nervous all at once. Holy cow, holy cow, holy cow. Luckily, I had just showered before we hung out with our friends, so I was feeling good and we were already packed. We got out our Bradley book (the birthing method we chose and had taken a twelve-week course in) to review what was ahead of us. We knew we'd be having a baby within 24 hours!

I called my parents and started to get my first contraction, just 10 minutes after my water broke. Josh hopped in the shower, and the contractions started to pick up. By the time Josh was dressed, we started timing the contractions and they were 5 minutes apart. It was so weird. They definitely hurt and were already lasting 50 seconds each. We knew since my water broke that if we called L&D they would want us to come in immediately, and since we were planning on a natural birth we wanted to wait and labor at home as long as we felt was safe.

I sat on the birthing ball and bounced and rotated my hips to try and stay relaxed and get her down. By midnight the contractions were easily 4 minutes apart or less and about 1 minute long. So we went ahead and called L&D, and they told us to come in. We packed up and headed out. I couldn't believe we'd be returning with our baby girl!

We arrived at L&D at about 1 a.m. The contractions did not slow down as I anticipated they might when you check in and get settled. They allowed me to be intermittently monitored, 20 minutes on, 20 minutes off. We walked around when I was off monitor, roaming the halls, and the contractions were very intense! They were about 2-4 minutes apart and 60-90 seconds long. Josh was an amazing coach, and we truly got to use our relaxation techniques and the breathing we learned in our Bradley classes. He would talk me through each contraction, and I was mentally able to completely go "somewhere else" (I was either on Laguna beach or at the top of the Eiffel Tower!) and of course I was praying a lot as well.

Funny enough, I kept having the song "Confidence" from the Sound of Music pop in my head. I kept thinking, "I have confidence in sunshine, I have confidence in rain . . ."

Ha ha. Also, we brought the birthing ball with us, so when we weren't walking I was at least on the ball. It was very helpful because it allowed me to move, as I knew I had to conserve some energy so I didn't want to walk every time.

Being monitored and staying in bed was horrible. I would have to lie on my side (lying on my back was even worse) and every time I contracted it seriously felt like my abdomen and hips and thighs were paralyzed. The only good thing was that I could see the contractions on the monitor, so it helped me to see when one was ending, and I would know I could make it through.

At 4:30 a.m. they checked me for the first time. They don't want to check you very often when your water has already broken, so as not to introduce the risk of infection. I was at 5 cm and 90%! I thought we were well on our way to Babyland. I continued to labor and it was very intense as the contractions built up and remained consistent. I knew if we could keep them coming I should be nearing transition by the time they checked me next time. They returned about 9 a.m. to check me . . . and I was still at 5 cm.

WHAT? Ugh. I couldn't believe it. They seemed surprised too, since my contractions were happening so consistently and were very intense but not progressing me. This started talk of Pitocin. I knew it would be extremely difficult to remain unmedicated if they intended on using Pitocin. I asked that we be given at least an extra hour to walk around and keep the contractions up and see if it didn't make a difference. They "didn't recommend" this, but we were going to do all we could to have a natural birth and didn't want to wimp out without even trying to continue this way.

So we went ahead and started walking (our nurse found us when it was time to get monitored.) Wow. What a painful hour! This time as I walked the halls with Josh, I literally had to stop every few steps. The contractions were less than a minute apart and lasting almost 2 minutes long and extremely intense by the time we got back to our room. They wanted to check me again and I just knew we had made progress.

My contractions were nearly on top of each other, and I asked to use the bathroom before getting checked. As I was in there the contractions would just not stop. I broke out in a cold sweat and then threw up (nightmare!) I was confused and shivering, and I knew these were all the telltale signs as Josh said to me, "I think you're in transition." I had to be. It was so horrible. But this was great news to me, because if I was in transition I knew we would have progressed and would be able to continue naturally.

I got to the bed and they checked me again. Still at 5 cm. No way. We couldn't believe it. We felt somewhat defeated, but at the same time we had told ourselves "Let's try the walking and if there's no change we'll know action needs to be taken." So after there was no progress again, we made the decision to get the epidural and have Pitocin started. I considered only getting the Pit, but I knew that if I wanted the energy to be able to push her out, I had no choice but to get the epi so I would be able to rest and regain some strength. I knew I wouldn't be able to endure it all without rest. Not after having been up for over 24 hours and in so much pain already.

I had endured 15 hours of completely natural labor, and I felt I had quite earned my gold medal for the day.

Getting the epidural was terrible in and of itself. They had to stick me three times because he said, "I'm sorry. Your joints are so close together I just keep hitting bone." (Which is just what you want to hear as they are putting a needle in your spine.) Ugh, as if I even wanted it in the first place. It was painful but tolerable until a contraction would come. Josh had been so supportive of me the whole time. He hadn't eaten or taken care of himself, so he nearly fainted when they gave me the epi! One minute he's there, holding my hand. The next thing I know, he's on the floor with his shirt off and they are giving him oxygen! Poor guy, he was white as a ghost!

Finally they got the epi, and after it took effect and they started the Pit I felt much better. Josh was able to sleep, and I was able to rest for at least a while. They kept saying they just needed to kick-start me and make sure my contractions were intense enough to keep me progressing and that I would have a baby by that afternoon. But the Pitocin was not progressing me. They decided to insert an intrauterine line that would measure the intensity of the Pit needed. The contractions were perfect, very often and very intense, but not progressing me.

Thank goodness, through it all, Matilda's heart rate

remained strong and steady. By 4 p.m. I was only at barely 6 cm. The clock was ticking, because it had been 18 hours since my water broke and they were concerned about infection. They were also concerned about the baby's position and size. We had known she would be big, and they were guessing about 8 lbs (which ended up being right!) Her head was transverse, and I had been rotating sides to get her lined up correctly. Also, she was only just now at -1 station. She didn't seem to be getting any lower and was possibly unable to at the angle she was. This is when the talk of a C-section became serious, and I knew it was truly inevitable.

We always knew it could come to this. I had prayed that God would make it very, very obvious and that we wouldn't be left with any other choice if that was what was supposed to happen. I had to just surrender it to God and believe that He was ultimately saving us from a dangerous route by backing us into a corner where a C-section would be best.

I was very grateful to have gotten to experience true labor! The water-breaking-going-into-spontaneous-labor experience was a true blessing I believe God let us experience since we had asked Him to let us have a natural birth experience. At this point, I felt like I was going into labor number three—natural, medicated, and now surgical.

It had been such a long day. We were emotionally exhausted and ready to just get this baby out. Within 20 minutes, we were in the operating room. It was very surreal, and I was feeling kind of woozy and trying to remain calm and keep my eyes open. I just wanted Josh by my side, so I was very glad to see him in his white zip-up suit and hat. (He looked like a hazmat worker!) Lots of pressure and tugging and pushing on my belly, and just minutes after that she was out!

Josh said later that she was so wedged in there the doctor had to move from one side of the table to the other just to maneuver her head out. Matilda cried, and we burst into tears!

She was here! She was ours!

It was magical and spiritual, and a rush of peace came over us. In the end, it turned out to be a huge blessing to have gone with the C-section. Afterward, in recovery with Matilda and Josh, I ran a 103+ fever. Turns out I was fighting off infection from having lost my water so long ago. My blood pressure and heart rate were up, and they started Matilda and me on antibiotics right away. They kept me on antibiotics the next 48 hours, and a day later my temp was finally normal.

It all worked out! I felt so blessed and truly not disappointed. I was really, really proud that I labored naturally for so long. Even though we had hoped for a natural birth, I stuck to my motto that "as long as you leave with a healthy baby (that's yours) that birth was a success!" And that is truly how I feel. Josh and I both cried when we made the C-section decision (both wrought with emotion and tiredness) but we knew as soon as we saw her it just wouldn't matter how she had arrived.

And it doesn't. We just LOVE HER!

And so it was with great joy and love we welcomed 8 lb, 8.5 oz, 22-inch-long Matilda Hazel Darling Pardy into the family at 5:03 p.m., November 1, 2009. Our darling had arrived! Praise be!

14

Welcoming a New Life (Mine!)

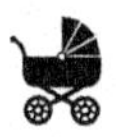

I had a daughter. A real live, wiggling little being with tiny fingers and toes cute enough to nibble right off her chunky little body. My eyelids were in a constant state of fight or flight as they wanted to slam shut from exhaustion yet remain open and staring at her beautiful face forever all at the same time.

Whose life is this? Mine. Who am I now? A mother. What time is it? It doesn't matter.

We were in a still-and-steady state of disbelief since hearing her first cry. But it was real. Here she was. And our hearts felt like they had gone through a strange, grinch-like explosion, growing "two sizes that day" and all the more with every minute we spent holding our new baby. It was impossible to have predicted this magnitude of love. I thought I loved my cat a lot. I knew I loved my husband immensely. I'd shaped my life around trying to love God with all I had. But never before had I felt such a deep, natural, impulsive, protective, and unconditional love as that which I felt for my child.

It seemed that there should be a whole new word a step beyond *love* just for babies. I kept using terms like *amazing*, *unbelievable*, and *incredible* and would find myself wincing at the incompleteness of their description. There are just no words for looking into the helplessly-wondrous eyes of your baby and sensing a new void in your soul that you are now able to tangibly hold in your arms. It was like staring at her and missing her all at the same time. I just couldn't imagine ever getting enough of her, ever.

Eventually something would break my trance, and I would be forced to tend to reality. Due to the infection and fever I had suffered, they kept me at the hospital an extra day. I always thought I would want to max out my time there, take advantage of the adjustable bed, the lactation consultant, and the nurses who smiled and seemed to know everything. But by the time our final night had come and those lovely nurses kept checking in every fifteen minutes or anytime the baby cried, I was ready to go home. Matilda was nursing well, and I was ready to sell my left arm in exchange for a hot shower and my own pillow. I longed for the comfort of the familiar and wanted to introduce Matilda to the world that awaited her.

But checking out of the hospital makes the dreamland of the birth experience come to a shocking halt. The daylight strikes you, and there you are—suddenly in a parking lot alone with your baby trying to figure out how to gently strap her into the giant car seat for the long ride home. This initial insecurity is your first test to conquer as a new parent. *If we can just make it home*, you think, *then I really think we can do this.*

You do. And you can.

CRYING, CASSEROLES, AND CLOCK-WATCHING

The first days at home are a blurry memory of crying, casseroles, and clock-watching. *When did she last eat? What time was it when she woke up? How long has she slept? And when can I take more pain meds?*

Recovery is hard. Harder than I thought. Granted, the doctor who discharged me told me that going through 19 hours of labor and ending in a C-section was "like running a marathon and then getting sawed in half." And it really felt like it. I'd watched enough *Baby Story* shows to know I wouldn't be doing cartwheels as I left the hospital, but still, the pain I felt was excruciating. It's difficult for me to manage my pain level. I know this about myself after having gone through multiple surgeries in my life.

While my pain tolerance is fairly average-to-high (I suppose you can't endure 15 hours of natural labor without some endurance) I tend to metabolize painkillers at a very high rate, which means I almost always need them sooner than when I can take them next. I had not been prepared for taking it as easy as I needed to. I didn't realize that slicing through multiple layers of stomach muscle wouldn't allow me to sit up or lie down without being helped. I was fairly anchored to my bed for a while, only getting up when I absolutely had to and grimacing when I did.

One night around midnight, I couldn't take it anymore. The baby was sleeping. I was down to one final dose of my painkiller, and I felt just awful. I burst into tears, worried sick that something might be terribly wrong inside my body. How was I supposed to know what felt normal? How could I endure any more pain? What did healing feel like and when would I be back to my old self?

So I did what any hysterical new mother does at midnight when they are in brutal pain—I complained to my husband until he convinced me to call the nurse. After all, that's their *job*. That's what they're there for. And you will not be the only hysterical mother calling them that week (or even that night, probably.) So get over yourself and just do it.

I will never forget that phone call. I was beside myself, trying to describe the pain to the nurse in between my whimpers. I remember asking, "What is a normal level of pain to expect at this point?"

And she very seriously and nonchalantly responded as if reading from a prompter, "You can expect to experience deep, burning pains that feel like a knife stabbing you in your middle over and over again."

"Oh," I said. "Well, yes. That is what I'm feeling."

She promised a refill of medication and wished me well and hung up. So there it was. Apparently my deep, burning, stabbing pains were entirely normal. And somehow, just knowing I wasn't crazy or at the brink of death was enough for me to grab a few hours of sleep before the baby woke up again. There was nothing anyone could say or do to help me heal any faster, really. Not that it stopped them from trying.

My mother had flown out just hours after Matilda was born. Since my labor initiated with my water breaking, it guaranteed a birth within 24 hours, so my mom quickly purchased a plane ticket and flew from Kansas to California in time to meet her new granddaughter before I even had a chance to sleep. It was wonderful and overwhelming and altogether surreal.

My dad flew out just a couple days later, and soon enough, our little apartment was a diaper-changing, breastfeeding, casserole-making, coffee-brewing machine in full swing. This plan had been determined long before my first contraction. It is hard to make a schedule around an event that has no predetermined date or time. The fact that both sets of grandparents lived out of state meant they simply couldn't be there as soon as we might actually need them. But the alternative to having them come out "around" the due date and wait didn't make sense to me either. Besides, I worked *right* up until the end and didn't want to give up any maternity time before the baby arrived in exchange for missing out after she was here.

My sister flew out for a few days after my parents left, and then Josh's parents arrived shortly after that and just in time for Thanksgiving. Not to mention, we were nearly the first of our young friends to have a baby, so there was always a slow trickle of visitors coming over to observe the pioneers of parenthood we had become.

Help is wonderful. Help is appreciated. Help is *necessary*. But help is not free.

Don't get me wrong. I don't mean your friends or family have any ill motives or any intention of hindering you or burdening you in any way. But visitors require consideration, and it is important to weigh values at such a sacred and fleeting time.

LIVING THE DREAM WITHOUT EVEN SLEEPING

My husband was thankfully able to take four weeks off work when Matilda was born. Before she arrived, we eagerly anticipated this time away from the office together. We had never taken more than a week off at the same time, so we looked at this upcoming leave as a glorified vacation. We dreamed of sleeping in late, snuggling our precious baby in between our smiling faces as we lay in bed, still in our jammies mid-afternoon. We envisioned sunlit mornings of coffee and breakfast that our friends would have lovingly dropped off as we rocked our cooing bundle of joy. We fantasized about strolling around the neighborhood, having people stop us just to tell us how adorable our daughter was and gasping when they noted how well we were doing, how well-rested we seemed, or how slim I already looked.

This illusion died quickly after we returned home from the hospital. It's one thing to joke about how the baby will keep you up at night. It's another to actually only sleep 90 minutes at a time for two straight weeks. You try to sleep when the baby sleeps or keep a smile on your face as your husband bounces her while she screams for you. You hate to ask your mother to please change the baby again or to reheat your coffee one more time, but you can't bear the thought of exerting the energy to do it for yourself. And you just want to be alone. Alone with your baby. Alone with your husband. Alone with yourself and your aching belly and your swollen breasts to just stop and breathe and take a sane minute to evaluate all the life changes that have happened within the last several days.

But there is no chance for being alone. Even trips to the bathroom come with guilt that you might be taking too long. Relaxing showers are hindered with calls questioning whether you are okay or if you need any help. And any sleep you do get is sprinkled with worry at every gurgle, hiccup, or coo that erupts from your baby's lips.

You want your baby all to yourself. You want to make sure that she knows you are the most important person to her, that she should need you and want you the most. You want to be the sole cure for her discomfort and the answer to her cries. You can't bear the thought of her need going unmet for even a second, so you find yourself changing barely-wet diapers and feeding her until she pukes and then worrying if you should start over or not.

You live in a constant state of *Am I doing it right?* and *I know best!* all at the same time. You want your parents to tell you what to do, but you don't want to take any advice either. You desperately wish you felt as confident as you seemed when you first held her in your arms, and you long for that moment when the world seems calm and right. And those moments come and go throughout each day.

The good thing about newborns is that God made them to sleep a little longer than normal in those first days. They just want food and warmth, and your chest offers both room and board for them. When your baby falls asleep on your body, resting all their weight and love on top of your beating heart, the world simply fades away. Your mother-in-law's advice becomes simply words. The dishes in the sink become easily-ignored clutter. A friend texting just to check in on you becomes background noise. This beauty in your arms is really all that matters. Keep focused. Stay the course. Remember this moment.

15

Making the Most of the Early Days

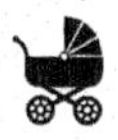

It's important to protect your time, energy, and memories in these early days. The first six weeks of parenthood are truly sacred. You will never get any time back in your life, but this particular allotment of days should be spent as if they are your last. Treasure them, guard them, and do all you can to enjoy them exclusively.

It seems entirely not fair to need so much help during a time when you just want to be alone. I don't have any regrets about having help and visitors and family join us in the first days of parenthood, but I wish I had known what to expect and how to kindly communicate my feelings more effectively (genuinely impossible on so little rest.)

You might need to ask your mother to be quiet. You might need to tell your sister to hand your baby back to your husband so he can hold her. You might need to tell friends to visit next week instead. You might need to order in every night for two weeks. You might need to cry every morning. You might need to tell your neighbors to turn their music down. You might need to ask your dad to leave the room so you can expose your breast and practice nursing again. You might need to turn your phone off for a while. You might need to ask your husband to hold the screaming baby so you can shower. You might need to ask your friends to do your laundry for you—even the stinky pile that is spotted with blood, milk, or baby spit-up. You might need to ask your visitors to leave early so you can sleep. You might hurt someone's feelings unintentionally. You might need to ask forgiveness from them when you get up from your nap. You might.

But all those things will fade with time, and your only chance for capturing these memories forever is if you set up some boundaries to allow for it. This is your time. This is your baby. This is your new life, and you are going to have to fight for it.

And sometimes you might even have to fight yourself for it.

SCARY TIMES AND SACRED DAYS

I had always been on guard for signs of postpartum depression. We've all heard or read the horror stories of mothers being blindsided with an eruption of emotions or an avalanche of insanity, and I didn't want to be unprepared in case something hit me. Besides, I had plenty of reason to carefully watch for red flags.

In my early twenties I had suffered bouts of depression that later were diagnosed as linked to hormonal imbalance along with a myriad of stressful circumstances. I'd spent a few years on the antidepressant Zoloft and in my fair share of counseling that had helped me to work through, pray, and fight my way to the surface of happiness and functional living once more. I knew my own triggers and signs of a spiral downward, and I knew that anytime there are great shifts or changes in lifestyle (good or bad) there is a chance for stress to turn into uncontrollable emotion.

It was only a couple weeks after bringing Matilda home that in the middle of the night I heard the first lies. My exhaustion and pain had left me in a vulnerable place, and if there were ever a time for spiritual warfare to sneak in and try to steal my joy, this was it. Call it hormone imbalance, call it Satan, call it insecurities at their worst, but a lie is a lie is a lie. I stared at my precious new baby, nursing her sweetly and thanking my God for the miracle I held in my arms . . . and suddenly a wicked vision of evil swept over my mind. In a moment, I nearly gasped out loud at my own thought. Did I truly have the capacity to conjure up the idea of hurting my own child?

No. Never. I would never ever do anything to harm this sweet baby.

The visions did not end there. Several more split-second attacks struck me over the following weeks. I would "see" myself smother my baby in my sleep or lose control of the stroller or drop a knife on her while I fixed dinner. It was gruesome. It was awful. It was very, very real. These thoughts turned into irrational fears. I worried that if I went on a walk and had an attack that I truly *might* lose control of the stroller or at least I worried that it wasn't worth the risk. So I stayed home. I began to distrust myself and my own instincts, silently embarrassed that I couldn't override my own emotions with the knowledge of reality and truth and prayer that weren't making these fears go away.

Worst of all, I felt great shame for having had the thoughts. Not that I dwelled on them or ever invented the ideas myself. I wanted nothing more than to silence these lies and move past the irrational fears and simply stroll my baby freely and cook dinner without worry. But how could I talk to someone without them questioning my true motives? How could I share these feelings without someone judging me or how much I truly loved my baby? How could I trust someone to believe that I would never harm my baby and yet couldn't stop worrying about the possibility of it happening?

More lies. It had to stop. My reliance on the truth became essential at such an irrational time. The truth was that I loved my baby. The truth was that I had friends and family who *knew* me, even if I wasn't sure I knew myself. And the truth was I needed a little help.

I came clean to my husband, my loving, trusting, wholly-understanding husband. We recognized these lies together and he helped me see that this was not from me, not from God, and not to be tolerated any longer. The shame I felt in keeping these fears secret was directly met with love and immediately replaced with relief and acceptance. Just getting the words out in the open, sharing them and recognizing them for the lies they were, almost entirely relieved the guilt and power they held over me.

I immediately sought counseling, and within a few weeks of sharing my fears and replacing my lies with loving truths the attacks were completely diffused. I consider myself lucky. Well, blessed really, I suppose. I didn't end up going back on medication or needing to continue counseling for long. I had a loving husband who supported me through a dark trial. I was able to function through the shadows and quickly regain my confidence and fully restore trust in myself and in my ability to care for my baby. But it wasn't without pain and effort and laying down my pride (even false pride is not easy to let go of.)

Postpartum depression has many forms. All scary. All unfair. All unpredictable.

You feel so many new emotions after giving birth that it can seem impossible to discern the normal from the unnecessary. You have to be ready to fight for what you want—your joy, sanity, confidence, and dignity. You have to recognize that Satan would love nothing more than to take these things from you, and you are in a vulnerable place for him to sneak in some insecurity wherever he can. You have to be willing to trust God when you can't trust yourself. Trust your character when you may not recognize who you are. Trust your relationships when you can't face your own identity.

Seek help and truth and love. Drive out the fears and lies. And rely on those who care for you. You are not a burden. You are not a bad mother. You are not supposed to know how to handle this. Allow time for healing and help. Pray like you've never prayed before. And don't stop holding that baby, rocking and staring and soaking up all the unconditional love he or she has to give you. Those early days are so precious, and no one can steal those moments from you. Don't allow it.

16

I've Got You, Babe: When Daddy Goes Back to Work

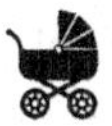

The four dreamy and chaotic-filled weeks my husband stayed home after Matilda's birth seemed to fly by at lightning speed. Before I knew it, he was picking out his shirt and tie for the next morning when he would abandon me and the baby to fend for ourselves (well, that's how it felt) and return to work.

On one hand, I was eager to get into a routine. I knew I could do this, right? I mean, as a nanny in my twenties I'd supervised multiple children all day long on my own. How hard could it be to care for one tiny infant? But this was *my* tiny infant. And it wasn't so much that I was worried about whether or not we'd survive the day. It was that we didn't want to survive the day without Daddy.

Daddy! How could we really enjoy ourselves if we couldn't all be together? How could he miss a smile or a smirk of hers? Heaven forbid he not be there to witness something new—a first giggle or wave! The thought of it was torture, and I kept contemplating how in the world we could make this work. Couldn't we all just live happily together and figure out how to work from home? Couldn't he just email all his work in from the comfort of home when the baby took her nap?

Sigh. I did not want him to go. We had just shared as much as two people could ever share, and here he had to go back to the world of cubicles and copy machines and miss out on the daily nuances of our little bubble.

The morning he had to go back was not my finest moment. I didn't want him to feel badly—I knew this was a necessary evil. No, not even that. It was a necessary *good*, but it wasn't as good as having him home. We had been living an illusion for the last month, and our bubble was getting burst at the sound of an alarm clock bright and early.

I tried to hold it in. I tried to keep calm and smile. I could feel my stomach in my throat as he bent down to kiss me and the baby, and we waved at the doorway as if sending him off to war. (God bless you, military wives out there who go this alone with your man fighting for our country. You have my wholehearted respect, and I'm in complete amazement that you are able to function, let alone take care of a child, after saying good-bye to your spouse on leave. My prayers are with you. Whew!)

I took Matilda back into the nursery to rock her back to sleep. I nursed her and wept. I let it go. The tears streamed down my face as I looked down at my sweet girl and thought, "Okay, here we go! Just you and me today, babe." I took a deep breath, snuggled her close, and thanked God for the last several weeks we'd had together living in our bubble. That season had passed. I had to stop and grieve the loss of the bubble, the loss of the dreamy time together, and allow room for what was to come in order to appreciate it fully. After all, my time was coming, and I wasn't going to let this grief trump my being able to make the most of right now.

THE TIME MACHINE

Josh's returning to work made the clock tick all the more loudly in my head. I had nine more weeks of maternity leave to soak up before *I* had to return to work. Tick tock. Tick tock. My baby was changing before my eyes, and I could feel the tears well up in my face at the thought of her going off to college and getting married next week. I'd expected the birth of my daughter to be a lot of things, but I'd never expected her to be a time machine.

Babies shove your life into warp speed. Those final weeks before birth are in such slow motion (waiting, waiting, waiting) that when the baby arrives, time has a lot of catching up to do. *ZAP!* That first week is a goner. While you are waiting for your milk to come in and your baby's umbilical cord to fall off, the rest of the world is zipping around you. You lose track of hours and can't tell anyone what day of the week it is.

Babies bring with them a strange, new perspective that allows us to see the future happening right in front of us all at once. You get glimpses of her growing up with each yawn she takes (so precious) or start to see which parent she looks like as she opens her eyes more and more (Daddy's girl) or begin to see her preferences as she reaches out for different toys (Ah, a giraffe-kinda gal. Maybe she'll be a zoologist or a safari guide some day! Oooh, blocks! Maybe she's gonna be an architect!)

It's fun to dream and speculate one minute and the next you are staring at that tiny face again, trying to memorize it and hoping the moment will never pass. But you can't pause time, as much as you try. You can't keep it all in your head, even if your eyes get watery and everything goes blurry because you just can't bear to blink and miss something. All you can do is saturate your mind with as much "present" as will fit and hope that it sticks.

Herein lies the paradox of the new baby.

YOU CAN'T HAVE IT ALL

You can't have her stay little *and* learn new things every day. You can't have her nurse forever *and* become independent. You can't have her keep you up all hours *and* be able to fully engage in every single moment of her new life with your complete attention. You can't. You're not (as far as I know) a robot or Jesus or drinking *that* much coffee to be able to keep it up. It's impossible.

And I hate it.

It feels irrational to our souls to live in a block of time. Our insides want to flip inside out when we look at our child, and we want them to hold still and never change. And we want to teach them everything we've ever learned and be there to see them grow old and change the world for the better. I think this particular feeling is sort of exclusive to parents (or at least I never felt it prior to parenthood) and I don't think it goes away once you feel it.

I first felt this paradox when I saw my daughter smile (really smile, not just gas) for the first time. I was at home alone with her, and I just couldn't believe it was happening. And then I just couldn't believe it was happening with no one else to see it. I was happy and sad all at the same time. I couldn't help but squeal with joy and then feel a little tear settling in the corner of my eye. I got to be there for it! I saw it! Her first smile! But it was slightly bittersweet to not have someone else there to see it too, to help me lock it into time forever, to share the memory of this moment for all time. And then the event had passed. All at once, as quickly as it happened (that sly, little smirk) it all disappeared in an instant and I was left with a quandary of emotions that seemed to tear a Grand Canyon through my heart.

This sounds dramatic, I know. When I listen to stories of other people's kids smiling or rolling over or pooping or clapping or whatever, I'm easily bored and slightly amused at best. I understand. You think you will handle this much more rationally. You think you will maybe Instagram the event, caption it, and email it to your relatives, maybe even post the YouTube video of it on Facebook for the world to see, and then you will happily move forward in life. Perhaps. No doubt there are plenty of times we distract ourselves with technology to literally upload our feelings for the world to validate.

But can we just admit that part of us does all that (the photos, the videos, the status updates) to try and cling to the present and have others jump into the moment with us so that it can all last just a wee bit longer? Maybe you can relate to this feeling after all. Maybe you already do this with your dog or cat or that fantastic meal you ate at that hip restaurant the other night. But when it is *your* baby you can multiply that feeling about a million times and start to get close to how you'll be feeling. Just ask any parent.

After my daughter smiled at me, I knew my perspective of how the world operated would never be the same. I knew I could never take enough pictures to keep her a baby forever. I knew I couldn't capture time and keep it at bay and let it play out as slowly (or quickly at times) as I would like it to. And to top it all off, I was really, really tired.

17

Embracing Motherhood One Cup of Coffee at a Time

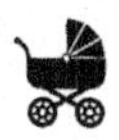

You don't know the definition of tired until you've had a baby. People, I'm talking *tired*. You might think you know what tired is like. Maybe you've pulled an all-nighter here or there, even had to work the next day or done it a couple days in a row. But back then, you only had yourself to consider. Now you have a little human completely and utterly dependent on you, fully relying on you and your short-circuiting brain to fire on all cylinders at every moment to meet their needs at all hours of every day. Forever.

The hardest part of bringing a new baby home is learning to function on no sleep. This is exactly why every parent tells all expecting couples to sleep as much as they can while they can. It's an envious time you won't get back for quite a while. The luxury to sleep when you actually need it is something you can't help but take entirely for granted. When you don't get enough sleep, you suffer emotionally, spiritually, physically, and relationally. God will give you enormous amounts of grace to keep going (seriously, I can't help but think the Holy Spirit is a heavily-caffeinated being Who especially helps us in our time of sleeplessness) but it's still not easy.

There will be a time you will want to scream and cry and sell your baby in exchange for a long nap. There will be a time when you want to hand her over and beg your husband to figure out a way to breastfeed her himself. There will be a time you will cry or eat or yell, not because you are feeling down or hungry or angry, but because you are so exhausted you don't know what else to do.

And just when you think you can't handle it anymore and you're going to suffer a narcoleptic episode in the middle of rocking your baby to sleep (while standing up) you will look down at that tiny, angelic face and never want to sleep again (though this may be the brain misfiring at three in the morning.)

Joy is funny that way. It hits us just when we need it most. And what is most frustrating about the lack of sleep is not the crazy emotions, not the crying baby, not the inability to focus on tasks or the short fuse you have with others. The most frustrating thing about being exhausted is being too tired to truly enjoy it all.

ZOMBIE PARENTING: HOW TO RAISE A HUMAN WITHOUT ANY SLEEP

I've always thought it was harshly unfair for God to give you this beautiful, uncaptureable, unreliveable time in life while you're relentlessly pooped. The sheer fatigue of caring for a newborn is hard enough. But to have the desire to engage with your whole mind, heart, and soul and not be capable of mustering the energy to do it is just cruel.

You can only do the best you can. Repeat this: *I can only do the best I can.* And this: *I am not a robot.* (Maybe don't say that last one out loud. Others might really think you've lost your marbles.)

It's sad and it's true. And if you don't believe it now, you will have an "Aha!" moment in the middle of the night when you're rocking your screaming bundle of joy soundly to sleep after singing "Jesus Loves Me" 800 times at four in the morning and finally collapsing on the bed, finding yourself torn between kissing your pillow and kissing your baby. You can't expect yourself to entirely grasp every new moment with your baby at 100 percent on only 50 percent of sleep. You will not only disappoint yourself and waste critical energy worrying instead of spending it on much more important things like smiling at your husband or combing your hair.

You've brought a new life home. *Your* new life. And you will never be the same. (This is a good thing!) Maybe you thought you would bring home a new human and remain unchanged. Okay, you didn't *really* expect to be unchanged. You thought you would grow a new capacity for love (you did) and potentially become more selfless (you are) and even feel closer to God (you will.) But now this baby is outside your body. You've become a mother. You might be taking less showers and changing more diapers, but the core of you is still the same. Right?

Or weren't you wanting a new identity when you decided to have a child?

Identity is a touchy thing. I sort of cringe every time I hear the word. Before I was a mother I would roll my eyes at women who would drone on about "feeling lost" or "losing myself" or not knowing "who I am" after having a baby. To be honest, I would think, "Get a grip, lady" and scoff at the idea that something so cute and small could dictate something so enormously esoteric as a person's selfdom.

Besides, I knew that my identity wasn't in having a baby. I learned through the long and heart-wrenching process of conception that I had to find my strength, hope, and future in God and not myself. I had come to a place of understanding through the pregnancy that I was not in control and that I was here to be more than just a gestational carrier for this child. So why was it shocking to me, now that the baby was outside of my body and I was the person chosen to be her parent, that I didn't want it to be all-consuming?

It did, in fact, consume all of me. This new baby ate up all my time and energy and still asked for more. She was insatiable. She was demanding. And I was happy (albeit, tired) to give in to her again and again and again. It wasn't sacrifice. It wasn't martyrdom. I loved her and was highly motivated to keep providing whatever she needed whenever she needed it.

Here is what the baby books won't tell you: It's okay to let your baby become your identity for a while. (Emphasis on the words *for a while*.) In this day and age, with all the identity crises and feminism and me-time and all those other buzz words that make sure we know it is okay to have a moment apart from our needy household, you rarely hear encouragement for the opposite.

Allow yourself to fall in love with being a mother. Fall in love with your baby as you stare at her during those exhausting middle-of-the-night feedings. Let yourself be utterly happy to just be in her presence, and revel in the contentment it provides for the moment. Cherish the "enough-ness" you feel in those times of being needed. No other role in your life will offer this same reward.

Why must we be immediately fearful of the possibility that all we will ever be is just a mother? Can we not appreciate the fact that to be only a mother is to be the entirety of somebody else's world for a small moment in time? I'd say to become someone else's complete universe, if for even a few short weeks, is the utmost of all identities.

Don't worry. The time will come when you are ready for more. You will have plenty of time to return to the world of the living and well-pedicured. Soon enough you will be shopping in Target or worrying about someone else's drama again. You'll be needed in another way for another reason by someone else before long. You will discover new talents you never thought you had.

The only thing your identity *isn't* is limited. Motherhood starts off as entirely consuming, but just as when you fell in love with your husband for the first time, it wears down and hits a comfortable rhythm that is manageable and peaceful (though forever unpredictable.)

Be a mother. Be all mother. Own it, enjoy it, and you will make it your own and do it unlike anyone has ever done it before. No one has ever mothered your child before. No one has ever been mothered by you before. Everyone is new at this and it's about to get real, real messy. Embrace it. This is who you are, and it is *so* enough right now. It's all you need to be.

Get some sleep. Practice smiling. And when you finish that cup of coffee, take a deep breath. We're about to stand in front of a mirror and finally dish on the subject you've been curious about ever since that baby came out—your body.

18

Body of Evidence

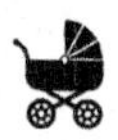

I've always thought it would be nice if when they send you home from the hospital with mountains of paperwork and pamphlets that they included a new road map for the postpartum body. Not instructions for recovery, but an actual brochure introducing you to your new skin.

Welcome to your new body! Have your boobs started leaking yet? Don't worry! Soon they will be engorged with fresh milk for your new baby and you'll be explaining to visitors what those wet splotches on your shirt are! Got that jelly belly? Have fun playing games with your new stomach like "Count how many jiggles on the car ride home!" Have your ankles swelled to twice the size of Vermont, more than they ever did in your pregnancy? Keep flip-flops in fashion year round with your new cankles or learn to knit extra-wide socks in time for Christmas! Your body is full of exciting new features including (but not limited to) lack of bladder control, zero stomach muscles, achy hips, swollen and/or cracked nipples, and possibly dozens of glorious new stretch marks (with maybe more to come!) Helloooo, mama! Isn't this the future self you always dreamed of?

Yikes.

The pregnant body came with certain expectations. Obviously, I knew my stomach would enlarge. I'd read enough books and talked to enough friends to get an idea about certain aches or pains that might come my way. My doctor and birthing class instructor had tuned me into the natural changes that were taking place and how it was affecting my growing baby.

But, let's face it, as far as I knew the postpartum body was pretty much a crapshoot.

During pregnancy, I had gotten used to the big belly, the strangers' hands drawn to it with eerie magnetism, and the bug-eyed glares from across the room from people who couldn't understand the walking miracle I had become, as my ginormous belly seemed to defeat all laws of physics. I had developed such deep appreciation for the wonder that was developing inside that I had somehow resigned myself to embracing this other-worldly body that seemed oddly familiar. I was in love with my unknown, unborn baby, so perhaps by default I came to adore the vessel that was protecting it.

But now that same vessel had come to the end of a difficult voyage, and the journey had left its evidence behind, much to the chagrin of the happy explorer (that would be me.) Did I travel an exciting adventure? Or had I shipwrecked myself helplessly beyond repair?

To be honest, prior to delivery I hadn't given much thought to my after-baby body. I suppose I was living in a little bit of denial, that somehow if I looked at enough *Us Weekly*s and *People* magazines that my thighs would absorb the idea of how to look or my abs would catch the drift that they couldn't remain hidden forever. But, the truth of the matter is, unless you have won the genetic lottery (I'm talking to you, Heidi Klum) your body will never, ever be the same as it used to be once you've had a baby.

Be careful how you interpret that last sentence. I didn't say your body would be *worse* than it was before. I said it would never be the same. And how could it be?

Are your emotions the same? Is your heart the same? Has your mind been altered or your soul changed or the lenses through which you view the world changed forever? Yes, of course. And we expect and hope for all these things to be tweaked and expanded and challenged from the moment we find out a baby is coming into our lives. Yet we cringe at the idea of our physical bodies being changed after this grand physiological feat.

It's not easy to look at yourself in the mirror naked. I'll speak for myself, anyway. It's not easy to look at *myself* in the mirror (though I'm going to bargain that you can relate to me on this one.) And I mean anytime . . . ever. It's been said that when men look in the mirror they immediately see what they like and when women look in the mirror the first things they spot are their flaws. I think that's generally very true.

Unfortunately this habit dies hard, and after months of hugging my pregnant belly in the mirror I had to stop myself from audibly gasping when I first saw my postpartum self staring back at me after the baby was born.

For one, I had a giant, fresh scar at my bikini line from the unexpected C-section. My breasts had become awkward cantaloupes, and my belly had become a spongy pillow of leather that I could no longer suck in on command. My face was my own (albeit, tired) but as I turned to observe the backside, my rear was nowhere to be found. Instead, a flat, fleshy rectangle had replaced my curvy bum, and it was official I was never going to be able to wear pants ever again. Okay, maybe not. But, still the "curse" of the ponchy-belly-no-butt-mom body had plagued my being and won, and I was left feeling confused and strangely selfish for wondering how this had all happened to me without my knowledge.

Why did I feel so bad? Wasn't it enough that I had a new baby to focus on? Shouldn't I just be thankful that everyone came out alive and healthy and not care so much about how I looked or how many stretch marks were left behind?

But I did care. I missed me, and I wondered how I would feel about myself as the weeks and months would go on. I wondered how my husband felt about my body. I wondered how I could keep from resenting my new baby. I wondered if other people said kind or judgmental things about me when they left our house after coming for a visit.

I wanted to get my body back after having my baby; this thought was true. But there was a new and central question I had been dodging ever since staring into my child's eyes the day she was born: *Is this body even mine anymore?*

THE LAND OF MILK AND HONEY

I always knew I wanted to breastfeed. I won't harp on the endless benefits of breastfeeding. People have valid reasons for not doing it, sure, but as far as preference goes there really are zero grounds for arguing against it. It's the best, and I wanted the best for my child. So I was pretty gung ho on making it happen.

I'll tell you this though—the thought of it freaked me out. I mean, we know these are my boobs we're talking about, right? Boobs which, up until delivery day, had been in the joint custody of me and my husband, who was a pretty huge fan of them. Breasts are sexual and seductive. We spend our whole adolescence praying for them to develop, our whole single life learning how to modestly flaunt them appropriately, and then our whole childless-but-married life using them to win arguments. Or something like that anyway.

But never, never before had I ever thought of my breasts as a natural resource supply to sustain another human's life. It's weird. A baby is going to be sucking on my chest? And we're supposed to believe it won't feel sexual or violating or gross in any way?

I focused on believing in the benefits of breastfeeding and how good and healthy it would be for my baby, but I certainly had my reservations surrounding the whole thing. Plus, let's be honest, how did it all even *work*? I had read the books, talked to friends, and even taken a class from a registered lactation consultant, and still the mystery remained.

I was dreadfully nervous the first time I breastfed my baby. I was in recovery, still shaking from the hormone crash the C-section had brought on. It wouldn't have mattered though. I'm sure I would have been shaking from nerves if I had delivered naturally too. I recalled all I had learned and read. I let the nurse help me. I thought a little prayer in my head and then said out loud, "Okay girl, here we go" and she latched on. Boom. Breastfeeding.

Lots of work followed. It took weeks of practice before my daughter and I were in sync with what position worked best or how much she could eat or how many dozens of pillows under what arm I needed to master this new art. But soon enough we found a rhythm that worked.

Really, honestly, I had it way easy when it came to breastfeeding. I know so many women who have horror stories about clogged ducts or trouble latching on and who spend months just trying to troubleshoot with a lactation nurse. But I'll say this—I've never heard a mother regret the work it took to breastfeed.

And it *was* weird. Crazy, fantastic weird. It feels like relief and awe and provision all at once. Just like when you are pregnant and you don't mind your tummy expanding or the discomfort of feeling a kick in your ribs or having to use the bathroom every twenty minutes, there is something about breastfeeding that feels recognizably right and incredibly foreign in one motion. But unlike the growing pains of pregnancy, the art of breastfeeding offers something unbelievably and instantaneously triumphant: a happy baby.

If you look into breastfeeding your baby at all, one of the first things you will learn is that your milk is made specifically and exactly for *your* baby, just as unique as he or she is. Not only that, but the action of feeding releases endorphins (yep, those "feel good" chemicals) that literally make a mother happy to be nursing. Is God insanely amazing, or what? He thought of everything!

Breastfeeding is a true gift. I immediately loved it. You always hear about the bond a mother and child create during the nursing stage, and there must be something to that. No doubt, if you are unable to breastfeed for a myriad of valid reasons, your touch and love and presence anchor just as great a bond between you and your baby. But having experienced the privilege of being able to nurse my baby, I can only attest to the joy I felt when I was the one able to provide—directly from my body—for the child I had birthed. It was awesome. It was beautiful. It was so much greater than any worry or doubt I had felt prior to doing so, and I was deeply grateful.

That being said, it was also incredibly demanding. Breastfeeding is a full-time job. On top of changing diapers being a full-time job. On top of burping the baby, putting her back down for a nap, rocking her, strollering her, bouncing her, giving her tummy time, bathing her, and—oh, yeah—time to feed again already.

Breastfeeding will consume your already-hectic-to-the brim day, especially early on. It may take you forty-five minutes to finally feed the baby, and then the baby will need to eat an hour later. Just when you think you have gotten it and the baby has started to doze off, she will wake up and need to nurse again. It's hard work and you'll be full of questions nobody seems to know the answer to since this is *your* baby and *you* are the mother.

Should I feed her again? Did she get enough last time? Will she spit up if I feed her more? Should I feed her more since she just spit up? Should I wake her up to feed her? Should I feed her before we leave or after we get there? What if she needs to eat in the middle of the trip? What if she needs to eat once we get there? Where should I feed her? How long should I feed her? Shouldn't she stop crying if I feed her?

And the list goes on. People can offer to burp her, change her, rock her, and soothe her. But for the most part (unless you are going to also bottle feed, which creates additional questions) you are the only one who can feed her. It's special. It's precious. And sometimes it's incredibly annoying and inconvenient.

The baby seemed to own my body—my breasts, anyway. It was clear in those early days that my once-sexy boobs had turned into proverbial feed bags for my new infant. If there was anything *less* sexy than a feed bag it was lost on me, so I felt a strange shift in my womanhood as I struggled with how to react. If only I could take off my breasts, hand one to my husband and one to my baby and call it a day. Crass, perhaps. Practical, absolutely. And my tired-beyond-all-reason self could no longer distinguish between the necessary and the sacrificial.

Was it a sacrifice to breastfeed and give myself to my baby? Was it necessary to let my husband still enjoy my body? Didn't I want both of these things anyway?

Breastfeeding comes with many learning curves, but the greatest one of all is how to balance the needs of many—including you. This is, after all, your own actual body still. Right?

After I had my baby, I wanted to get my body back. I just didn't think it would be so literal. I'm not just talking about my ponchy belly or my saggy boobs. I'm talking about shrugging my shoulders up so tensely that nobody could touch me and cringing back at the thought of one more little finger poking my flesh with a request for fulfilling a need. Any need. They aren't being selfish, that crying baby or longing husband of yours, they are just being, well, *them.*

And *you* aren't being selfish for wanting to be left alone sometimes. It can feel unexpectedly invasive to be needed and pulled in so many different directions even when you sincerely want to be pulled in those directions! I wanted to feed my baby and I wanted my husband to desire me, but I couldn't tear myself in two. After all, it wasn't like I wanted to go from feeling like a Victoria's Secret model to a milk truck driver, but some days that is pretty much what it felt like. Nobody had told me what to do with these feelings or how to cope with them. All I could do was try and try and try again.

Try to be reasonable. Try to explain. Try to be fair. Try to be honest. Try to be a servant. Try to be humble. Try to feel the enormous amount of love that was being offered to me.

The "battle of womanhood" became a new and seemingly permanent storm. I wanted to be it all. And I wanted to be really super awesome at it. I wanted to be known for being really super awesome at it all. But all three of me (wife, mother, and individual) were going to have to learn to get along and get through this together and develop a way to rock the planet as an integral trifecta that couldn't be one without the others. (You getting this?)

This profound trifecta idea is what my boobs taught me, thank you very much, in the early months of motherhood. Breastfeeding was so much more than an experience with my baby; I was discovering a whole new self. A self that could give. A self that was thoughtful. A self that, as ironic as it sounds, was becoming more and more self*less* each day.

19

The Naked Truth

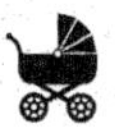

Selfishness is altogether strange. We know from the Word of God that genuine, real Christ-like love is not self-seeking (1 Corinthians 13:5 says just that.) We are warned against selfish ambitions and self-serving motives and manipulations, all leading to a path of destruction. We've all had personal experiences of feeling disappointed by someone who acted selfishly against us or we've even felt the conviction of having learned a lesson too late by hurting someone else's feelings because we chose our needs over theirs. It's simple but incredibly impacting, even when we find it impossibly difficult to abide by—selfish behavior is sinful, bottom line.

Then we have reality. We live in a nation where we are bombarded with magazines, television, social media, apps, tweets, and all kinds of insta-feelings being thrown our way about how we, we, we need this or that or have got to be getting such and such. You know, normal, every-day life centering around—who else?—me. Me, me, me. The reality we live in is self-centered. Self-seeking. Self-serving. Self-motivated. Give *me* what is convenient for *me*. Tell *me* how *I* can feel better. Let *me* know how *I'm* doing and so on. You get it.

These were the thoughts running through my head when I was standing in front of the mirror naked, wondering where I (the real me, that is) had gone. Who is *me*? And why did I so desperately want her staring back at me all of a sudden?

I fear selfishness. When I die and my family and friends are nibbling on casseroles and sipping coffee at the reception after my funeral, the last thing I would ever want anyone to say (or think) about me would be that I was a selfish person. Can you imagine?

"Boy, she really made time for herself, didn't she? I mean, her nails always looked grrreat!"

"That girl could always take such a long nap. She could pace the aisles of a store unlike anyone I've ever known. No doubt she's up in heaven relaxing just like she always did. She sure knew how to distract herself from accomplishing productivity!"

Recognizing this about myself, I had to be honest with God and seek a solution. 1 John 4:18 spells it out simply: "There is no fear in love. But perfect love drives out fear."

The only remedy to fearing selfishness is the love of Jesus. If I was going to seek a new self, I had to be completely willing to allow the full-and-perfect love of Jesus to transform me from the inside out. Again. And again and again and again.

TIME TO TAKE A SELFIE

This is when the Selfish Scale came to mind. It seems to me that as we live in a selfish world there must be some degree of change we are capable of with our own will. I know what you're thinking—*I'm not entirely selfish! I just donated to a charity in Haiti and cooked dinner for my family without any thanks! I just served in the children's ministry and gave my friend a ride to the airport!* Hurrah! You're right. We can choose unselfishness. We can see a cause greater than our own needs and fight for those who need help. We can be unselfish. We can go out of our way. We can lay down our expectations and give freely without wanting anything in return, and we can consciously make an effort to be kinder, gentler, and more compassionate to those less fortunate than ourselves.

But then what? Aren't we still left looking in the mirror wondering who will pat us on the back? Aren't we empty from giving so much that we eventually start to resent those around us for invalidating our sacrifice? Unselfishness looks good and can temporarily feel great. But our world is broken, and unselfishness is futile without an ultimate healer.

Go deeper. Selfish . . . unselfish . . . self*less.*

Selflessness is then the goal. We cannot achieve selflessness by ourselves. In fact, that's the whole idea. Selflessness requires nothing of us beyond our faith. Selflessness is purely acceptance that the love of God (so insanely more powerful than our own love) is going to flow through you.

Maybe it looks something like this:

Selfishness	**Unselfishness**	**Selflessness**
Me	My Ideals	Jesus
Fear	Functioning	Freedom

There you have it. I had to stop pursuing unselfishness, take it to the next level, and start fervently seeking selflessness. I had to start being real with myself about how God viewed me, what that felt like, what that looked like, and how that translated onto my husband and new baby. After all, how could I begin to love them (even on the most fundamental levels as sex versus breastfeeding) if I couldn't come to terms with how I felt about myself? I was an untrustworthy source. I couldn't tap into fickle-and-fleeting feelings anymore. I had to face something much greater and truer and more dependable—my Jesus.

Okay, Jesus, have at it. What do you think of my naked body?

Have you ever asked Jesus about this? Maybe not. Maybe this thought is no big deal to you. But for me this question was sort of terrifying. It even felt kind of inappropriate or shameful in some way. But those were my feelings getting in the way of truth again, not reality.

Why was it so uncomfortable for me to ask my Creator to tell me about myself? Shouldn't I have turned to Him in the first place to figure out how to feel?

I prayed. Naked, unashamed in the eyes of God, asking my Creator to tell me what to think about this body of mine. I'd spent so many years of my life trying to live up to certain standards, almost always letting myself down by not looking a particular way or being happy with certain aspects that were too large or too small or too cellulite-y or too saggy. Now, as a new mother, I recognized even less of myself. I had spent so many years listening to my own voice, telling myself how I felt and critiquing my body so constantly that I wasn't even sure I could hear what God had to tell me. Would I be able to distinguish truth from the lies I had come to know so well? It was certainly worth pursuing.

It didn't happen all at once. I didn't stand in front of the mirror naked one morning and walk out of the bathroom with a new kick in my step. I didn't put on Jesus goggles and look at myself like I was a Sports Illustrated model all of a sudden. It just doesn't work like that, and I don't want you getting any grand illusions that if you say a prayer and strip down to your skivvies you will magically fix all your insecurities. I wish.

But the process had begun, and that was something. The process toward truth. The process toward selflessness.

I went from staring at myself in the mirror to holding my new baby and staring at her beautiful little frame, her sweet smirky smile, her teeny tiny eyelashes that curled up in the corners. She was total. She was absolute. She was just exactly who she should be, and I couldn't imagine her any other way.

Spark!

The ignition of truth about my body had just turned over and fired up a spark of new knowledge within my being. Jesus looked at me the same way I looked at my daughter. Total, complete, and entirely sufficient to carry out the life He laid before me. Just. Right.

I had spent so much time worrying about whether my outsides were meeting my own needs that I had never stopped to consider that my body is already entirely complete to meet God's needs. My body was not my own. It never had been. And it took a baby physically demanding me in order to realize that I had always been a vessel, long before I carried a fetus to term and birthed a new human. Here I was, finally realizing I had been birthing things all along, completely unaware of their presence or impact. Gifts, miracles, sin, love, hate, apathy, empathy, and everything in between.

My body had been delivering truths and untruths according to how I allowed God to work through me. This is the process of how we choose between selfishness, unselfishness, and selflessness, all based on how closely we are listening to the truth of God. We are constantly motivated to act, but what motivates us and what we choose to listen to is going to make all the difference in how we decide what action to take.

THICK THIGHS AND BIG FAT LIES

Take a deep breath, maybe a sip of coffee. I know what you're thinking: *What does this have to do with how fat my thighs are?*

Everything.

We live in a world of input/output. In goes the coffee, out goes the energy. In goes the encouragement, out goes the confidence. In goes the insecurity, out goes the worry. It stands to reason that after years of feeding myself lies about my body I had become familiar and comfortable with insulting myself, expecting less, maybe even chronically living in disappointment with how things might age, especially after having a baby. The pregnancy had revealed to me a new appreciation for my body, but when you are looking in a mirror with saggy skin staring back at you it's difficult not to slip back into old habits.

What had I been putting into my body all these years? And what had it brought me? Maybe I thought that complaining about my body would bring me relief, perhaps even a little justification that it wasn't my fault or something. But it didn't. It just made me feel worse. That seems to be one of Satan's favorite tricks—slipping lies into your head through your very own voice, so much easier to swallow, as if we came up with the idea all by ourselves.

I needed new input, but what I really needed was extraordinary output.

20

Old Habits and New Hope

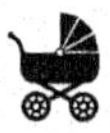

Maybe you're thinking I'm going to tell you how to change the tape player in your head or how you should recite verses or positive meditations over and over until you start spewing butterflies. I'm not. I think it is wonderful to tell yourself truths and positive statements, but relying on yourself is what got you here in the first place, so it seems silly to follow the same instructions and expect an entirely different outcome. That is the definition of insanity, isn't it?

So if we aren't going to be the source of input, we must turn to output. This, we have a choice about. What *action* can I take (regardless of what I'm currently feeling) to ensure a reliable and trustworthy input?

Let me state this in a way that makes more sense: Fake it till you make it.

This method of realigning old habits is underrated. Maybe it feels disingenuous at first. But let's think about it a second. Is it disingenuous when you are authentically and honestly making the choice to seek sincere selflessness?

Is it fake of me to choose to smile at my baby and love her in the middle of the night and go to her and feed her willingly, against all my natural feelings of wanting to sleep or resenting the fact that my husband isn't offering to make a bottle? Is it faking it to instead prayerfully pursue the selfless act of giving without expectation?

No. It's not fake to allow Jesus to take over, but it might feel unfamiliar. And it should. After all, I was done reacting. My natural reactions only led to selfishness and guilt. So it definitely felt strange and unnatural the first time I didn't make my husband feel guilty for snoring through the baby's cries in the night. I let it go. I didn't mention it in the morning. I rose above my natural response through the grace of God, and I chose Jesus instead.

And a funny thing happened. Out of this output came input. Not through my voice, my thoughts, or my ideas. Input comes in (duh) from the outside. And slowly, little by little, my actions were reaping wonderful benefits I had never expected.

My husband began to thank me for my patience. He complimented me on my perseverance with the screaming baby. He encouraged me in front of others and even praised my fortitude. He was a wonderful husband to begin with—I hadn't felt like these things were necessarily missing from our marriage. I was beginning to rely more on Him and less on me. This idea seems so basic, but it's incredibly difficult to live out in a real world, especially on very little sleep.

I think I was afraid that if I became entirely selfless no one would look out for me. I was worried that my boundaries would be lost and my guard would go down and my entire protection system would be disarmed. I thought I would get taken advantage of and that others would walk all over me. These are *not* things to pursue, nor are they characteristics of Jesus. Be careful and prayerful that you don't stumble into martyrdom in your search for selflessness. It will entirely defeat your journey.

SELFLESS STEPS TOWARD SANITY

True selflessness is a consistent choice you have to be willing to make in order to be more like Jesus. Just like love. Just like respect. Just like hope and courage and goodness. You must choose it beyond yourself and act on it regardless of your feelings.

You are not a victim. It is not sacrificial of you to allow your husband to sleep through the cries of your baby. You are sleep-deprived and cranky and don't feel well, and your natural instincts kick in to want to survive and shout your needs from the rooftops. And you have a great need. A spectacular need. An unimaginable need! For Jesus. Nothing more.

The beauty of pursuing selflessness is that, ideally, when we are all pursuing Jesus and trying to meet the needs of others in a healthy and reasonable way, our needs are completely met as well. This is the perfect design of relationship that Jesus created. The more we give of ourselves and put others before ourselves, the more Jesus that person encounters (less you, more Jesus) and the more motivated that person will be to reciprocate in a healthy and loving way. Output, input. Input, output.

Our marriage took on a new habit, a new cycle, a new passion for pursuing the needs of the other and the needs of our new baby. Soon I wasn't thinking about how much I "wished he would do such and such" a certain way with the baby. I wasn't focused on how much "me time" I wasn't getting. I wasn't feeling resentful for not sleeping or torn between who wanted my breasts more.

YOU'VE EARNED THOSE STRIPES

My body was not my own, but it was mine to freely give. It became a privilege, not an obligation, to allow myself the pleasure of giving. Blessings started to replace frustrations, and tension was diffused by shifting my focus away from myself.

And those thighs of mine? Well, maybe pursuing Jesus doesn't change the number on the scale, but I will tell you it genuinely has a slimming effect. As I study my stretch marks in the mirror, I can see so much more than ugly lines.

I'm not saying you will look at your body and not want to change something. It is still normal to want to improve yourself, to become healthier, or to look nice for yourself or your spouse. It's not unhealthy to want to feel pretty. God made women beautiful, and he made men attracted to our beauty. It is lovely and motivating to want to remain appealing.

But when I stopped and asked Jesus to tell me about this body of mine, I started to look at it differently. Those stretch marks had a story. This one is a battle scar that reminded me of how long I labored. This one helps me recall the wonder of the miracle that grew inside my belly. That one shows just how taxing it was to carry such a big baby for so long. And they all force me to remember how, for nine long months, God worked and developed an entirely new creation in this vessel so that she can one day make an impact for His kingdom with another purpose in another time for another reason. And I got to be part of it. I was there from the beginning of her beginning. These are not ugly scars; they're remarkable traces of impact. God has used me tangibly in the mark of His influence on this earth. Whoa.

If I had to bear a few stripes in the course of this occurrence, so be it. If my body changed because I had been part of such an extraordinary experience, I could more than accept that. I could choose to love it.

The depth of this revelation is easily lost. It only takes one good pair of cute, skinny jeans to send my mind into temptation towards forgetting everything I just said. We can sit and stare at our naked bodies and thank God for them every day, but if we can't zip up our favorite skirt, it can be really difficult to find confidence in the real world.

I get it. I understand these transcendent states of prayer can suddenly go flying out the window when we find ourselves rushing out the door with nothing to wear.

In all practicality, the postpartum body is difficult to dress. We've fought the mental battle—the bigger battle, mind you—but we're still left with the real-life quandary of clothing and events and trying to look and feel our best in front of everyone else. It's one thing to feel confident in front of Jesus, but it's another to step in front of judgmental gazes and maintain the idea that we are "just right" and totally acceptable.

21

Finding Comfort in the Uncomfortable

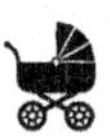

Every woman is different. Every body is different. You will absolutely meet someone who loses all their baby weight within a couple weeks of birth. You will also know someone who has yet to lose those last 30 pounds, and her baby is now packing a suitcase for college. Guaranteed, both those women have felt the exact same pressure to look a particular way within a particular amount of time after having had their babies. Is this not ridiculous?

After Matilda was born, lots of friends came to visit. Since we were one of the first among our friends to enter into parenthood, the visits came with much awkwardness and enthusiasm. Of our friends, the girls were usually giddy to hold the newborn, while many of the guys would shrug and wave off the offer as if they were avoiding the plague. They were overly complimentary and sometimes a little too honest. It's okay. It was all new for everyone really, so the initial grace extended and everyone left feeling a little silly but happy all the same.

That being said, when energy is running high regarding a life-changing event (wedding, death, birth) whether good or bad, people often aren't sure what to say. Again, that's okay.

Under this umbrella of grace, I tell the following tale: One of my husband's friends came to visit us. We were all close, and being the transparent people that we are, we welcomed questions anyone had about the birth, the delivery, or the insanity that new parenthood had thrown us into. I can't help it, then, that this friendly fellow responded honestly with a rather loaded question directed at me. "So, how long will it take you to lose all the weight?"

He's lucky I didn't punch him in the face; I'll tell you that much. If I hadn't known this question was stemming from an honestly inquisitive heart, I'm pretty sure I would have ripped his tongue out of his mouth right there. Okay, maybe not. But still, you should choose your words wisely around a hormonally charged and emotionally unstable new mother who is acutely sleep deprived.

Nevertheless, I was speechless. I think I finally fumbled out some gibberish about how it had taken me a good nine months or more to pack it on so it wasn't going to come off overnight, but whatever I said really didn't matter. I'm sure he shrugged and took the information into inventory for a later date when it would apply to the mother of his own children. But, to me, the words hung in the air like little balloons of expectation. He might as well have said, "Why are you still so fat?" because that's exactly what it felt like, intention or not.

And, honestly, I kind of felt the same way. Before I had entered into a conversation with Jesus about it, I had my own questions for my body. *Listen, body, you've had the baby! Snap to it! Suck it in! Lift, lift, lift!* I nearly picked up pom poms to cheer my muscles into regrouping themselves back into proper formation. To no avail.

WEIGHTING ON THE BABY WEIGHT: HOW LONG WILL I LOOK LIKE THIS?

Grace, grace, grace.

The mirror is rarely gracious to us. Our clothes are more often reminders of what doesn't fit than what does. The expectations we have of ourselves have more to do with what we see than what we know. And it's altogether unfair.

Grace, grace, grace.

Jesus invented grace and is never lacking in it. We need only turn to Him when our cup runs dry and our Spanx don't fit. So many times we measure our worth by the amount of granulated sugar we ingest rather than the grains of grace we take in.

The postpartum body requires grace. This is exactly why I began this talk from the inside out. Quality undergarments and a good concealer under the eyes will only get you so far. You might fool your friends into thinking you've taken back your smaller closet or your prepregnancy clothes, but none of it does any good if you can't grasp the worth that lies beneath it all.

You might need to realign your expectations. You might need to stop opening magazines. You might need to avoid supermodels on TV or anything else that might trigger you to cringe at the thought of your own skin. Remove the temptation if you must and reread the steps for pursuing selflessness to encourage the journey away from yourself.

It was a while before I felt like I was really ready for the public. Ever since my husband went back to work after the baby was born, I felt the clock ticking over my head. I knew my time was coming and I would need to splash back into the pool of reality, and from where I stood, that water seemed very cold and murky.

Not only did I feel like I didn't fit into that world anymore, but I barely fit into the clothes that I would have to wear to work there. "Business casual" they called it. It might as well have been a bikini with the discomfort it brought to my mind.

Was I ready for the public? Could I take the plunge with confidence and survive the sharks that might await me?

Before I could think about going back to work, I had to entertain the idea of just getting out. This is an essential step in the beginning of motherhood. It's part of reestablishing the new normal and reclaiming a routine that will help you to make the necessary transition.

You have to leave the house. With the baby. By yourself. In real clothes.

If you haven't had a baby yet, you are probably laughing at the serious tone to this idea. You might have grand illusions of strolling around happily and carefree, baby in tow and skipping along pleasantly. But if you've recently had your baby and you are reading this in between sessions of nursing or you are snuggled up in your cozy bed with your jammies on, the idea of leaving the house might terrify you.

Indeed, there is a first time for everything. You just have to do it.

Before I took this step, I too had grand ideas. I had loads of experience with babies in a safe and controlled environment. But never before had I gone out into the craziness of the unpredictable world and brought with me the ticking time bomb that was my very own little bundle of joy.

I immediately had a zillion unanswered questions. I never had thought to ask any of my friends or siblings or doctors about how to go about avoiding disaster on an outing with my newborn. After all, I didn't want to seem incapable or inept or silly or stupid or overly worrisome. I just figured everyone else must have known better than I did or read some book I hadn't or somehow had one extra mother-nurturing gene that I lacked.

But I did it. I put on uncomfortable jeans that didn't really fit. I put on a shirt that still showed wobbly belly underneath. I put on makeup while the baby wailed in her car seat as she waited for me. I tied shoe laces over my swollen Hobbit-like feet. I loaded her in the car and we drove to Target for absolutely no reason other than just to leave the house.

Within the hour, I found myself nursing my baby in the backseat of my Sebring way back in the corner of the Target parking lot, wondering if this was such a brilliant idea after all.

Is this what people did?

Evidently.

Sometimes, you just do what you need to do. My baby was hungry and I fed her, end of story. There would be future Target trips, trips that included massive poop explosions and purchases of new clothes out of necessity, losing favorite toys and rerouting the entire store with a screaming child until that toy was found, spitting up in an aisle so much that it required a mop-up job by a very cranky khaki-pants-red-shirt-wearing employee. Whew. But it all started with one little unsettling outing that gave me just the boost I needed to know I could conquer the world.

Okay, maybe not the world. But I could conquer Target, and that was enough for one day.

And you know what? It totally didn't matter what I looked like. The confidence boost I needed didn't come from my thoughts or the size of my jeans or even the compliments of others. My new-found confidence was sprouting from little seeds of truth and obedience and all the love and effort I was able to happily invest into this new life I so enthusiastically wanted to grow into a beautiful life.

The time would come for skinny jeans. The scale might *never* show me what I wanted to see. The years ahead would grant me the grace and time I needed to appreciate what was in the mirror. But the inside of me—well, that had changed forever.

I had grown a new human, developed out of a zillion cells and molecules and atoms that were strategically and perfectly placed in an order that only God could masterfully direct, and yet I was the one who felt new all over. I was the one living in new skin.

And it was about time to see what this new life was really made of.

22

Countdown to Returning to Work

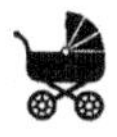

It was time to go back to work. Well, almost.

In the weeks leading up to the final date of my maternity leave, I felt like the giant clock that had been hanging over me for the last twelve weeks was slowly crushing me one inch at a time. It was no longer peacefully hovering like a rain cloud; rather, it was like a giant bag of bricks that weighed on my shoulders, gaining new bricks every day and getting heavier by the minute.

About three weeks before the big day, the tears came. I stopped in my tracks at the thought of leaving my little, bitty baby in the care of someone else. My brain no longer had the capacity to contain the notion, and it burst out of my eye sockets in the form of a flood. I sobbed. I ugly-cried. My shoulders rattled up and down and I made weird, guttural sounds as I gripped my baby girl against my chest and wept. I was sad. I didn't want to leave her. I couldn't imagine it, and yet I had no choice.

This may seem dramatic. I'll admit I was even surprised at how coreshaking the reality was becoming. I wouldn't have guessed I would be such a mess, especially when things had worked out so well for us. Our situation was pretty ideal, as my sister-in-law was going to be caring for our new baby while I was at work. It was the perfect setup, really.

After weeks of checking out daycares, worrying about finances, and trying to figure out all the logistics, our situation had become one enormous win-win, as we needed the help and she needed the money. Josh's amazingly-wonderful sister and her toddler daughter would come to our home, ensure the happiness and survival of our little Matilda, and I would be free from worry all the live-long day. Whew.

How I wish it had been that easy! While ideal, it was not worry-free. Don't get me wrong, I was incredibly thankful for our arrangement. I knew many moms who begrudgingly shelled out a lot more cash to heartwrenchingly drop off their child at a daycare. It was an amazing blessing to be able to leave our baby in the familiarity of her own home and in the hands of a sweet relative. But it wasn't me. And I wanted it to be me.

So I cried.

Many moms choose to return to work. Many moms love their jobs. That is wonderful for them, but I was not one of those moms. I had to work. We ran the numbers about a billion times, and the fact of the matter was that there was simply not enough money coming in with one salary. It wasn't just the money but the health insurance too. At the time, Josh and I worked at the same university, so we got a huge insurance break being able to combine our stipends. Yep, the math was simple—for the time being, I simply had to return to my job.

It wasn't that I hated my job. Most of the people were lovely, caring folks. The tasks I had were somewhat fitted to my gifts, and I had had enough terrible jobs in the past (thirty to be exact, but who's counting?) to know that this position as a video production coordinator at a Christian university was a title of privilege. I didn't want to be ungrateful. I just wanted to stay home and love on my baby!

I had just gotten used to having her in my life. Three months of building a little routine all our own—change her, feed her, take a nice stroll to Starbucks, feed her again, walk home, feed her some more, nap with her, play with her, feed her some more, maybe call a friend, play some more, possibly run to the store, feed her, cook some dinner, greet Daddy when he got home from work. Ahhh, it was precious.

I had some magical moments of strolling and sitting and staring at my baby, soaking up this new season of my life and feeling like time had stopped just for me and my baby so we could relax and take it all in for a moment. I remember sitting on a park bench on a cool winter morning (cool is about as bitter as winter mornings get in California) and Matilda had just fallen asleep in the stroller. I sipped a latte and wrote in a journal, and I couldn't imagine life getting any sweeter than that very second. I remember thinking right then if I could relive any moment, surely this would make my top five.

The simplicity of it all brought me great joy. I felt a freedom I had never felt while I was at work under the authority of someone else's watch. I got a taste of the life of a stay-at-home mother, and I liked it. Granted, those first few months with a newborn who is immobile and napping often are a lot more wondrous and a lot less time-consuming than the coming months would be. Still, it was a dreamy time and a wonderful illusion to live in for a short while.

HI-HO, HI-HO! DO I REALLY HAVE TO GO?

Tick. Tock.

It was the day before I had to go back. I laid out my clothes, confident that my final chosen outfit would be both slimming and comfortable for my first day back on the job. No doubt I would be feeling the eyes of many as they recognized me, including those oblivious to the fact that I had been gone for the last several weeks. I joked with my husband that I would just start telling people I had been at fat camp and look at them cock-eyed when they asked how the baby was. *What* baby? And then I'd laugh at them when they tried to back-pedal and salvage such an awkward moment. Ha!

Kidding aside, I was truly worried about people asking me about the baby. I honestly didn't know how I would react. Would I burst into tears at the mention of her name? Could I hold it together long enough to actually make it through the day?

I had a good, long cry the night before. I wanted to get it all out of my system so that I could wake up refreshed and focused. I had a big day ahead of me, and I needed all the energy I could muster.

Katie and her daughter, Sofie, got to our house bright and early. We all planned way ahead of schedule to ensure we could make it on time. I was still nursing, too, so I really wasn't sure whether to pump right before I left the house or to finish feeding the baby and head out. It was all uncharted territory, and nobody seemed to know exactly what to do.

We quickly reviewed any final details (I had already prepped Katie in an overly-protective-mother sort of orientation prior to her first day) and said our final good-byes. I gulped and kissed her cheeks. I left lipstick on each side of her face, and it made my heart sink at the thought that I had left my final mark on her for the day. Sigh.

Honestly, you would have thought I was going away for a month or more, the way my hands shook at my final wave. It was altogether overly drawn out. I'm sure my husband and sister-in-law were thinking, "Get a grip, woman! She'll be fine!" But I totally didn't care. They were extraordinarily patient and sympathetic with me. I was grateful to be able to wear my heart on my sleeve that day, as it felt like I was leaving part of my soul at home and going off to war.

The door shut. She would be okay. I would be okay. We could do this.

I felt much better by the time I arrived at work. I had only teared up a little but not even enough to run my mascara, so for that I was incredibly proud. I downed my travel mug of coffee and slowly climbed the stairs to my department, carrying a small box of new pictures I would proudly display in my cubicle.

Deep breath. I was back.

Everyone was very kind. All the guys said something like "Oh, you're back" while all the women tilted their heads in sympathy with a much more somber "Aww, you're baaaack." It was nice to be seen and appreciated, nevertheless.

Then the questions started. "How is the baby?" "How are you doing?" "Who is watching her?" "Do you have any pictures?"

I could nearly feel my bottom lip quiver at each new inquiry. It was not easy. While I was grateful for the interest, I couldn't help but cringe with guilt anytime anyone brought up the subject. Not just guilt, but sadness.

I missed her! I was missing *out* on her! I was grieving the end of a wonderful era, not celebrating my grand return to a job I hadn't missed. I wanted somebody to come up, hug me, and just say, "I'm so sorry you have to be here! Let's go punch someone in the face and eat some chocolate!" because that's about all I felt like doing.

I'll say it—I felt sorry for myself. I had grown up spoiled by the convenient notion that once you had a baby you magically got to stay home and relax. Even though I had known before I ever even got pregnant that I would need to return to work in order to support the family, I was mad that it hadn't all worked out as easily for me.

I became jealous of friends who got to stay home with their kids. I was jealous that my husband was able to focus on a task without feeling guilty and, most of all, I was jealous that someone else got to spend all day with my baby. Honestly, I hated it. And I began right then and there, sitting at my cubicle and staring at my computer monitor, praying that God would allow me the freedom to live and learn in this unwanted phase.

I knew I couldn't just drag myself into work every day, leaving my heart at the doorstep of my apartment and constantly worried that my baby would begin to prefer the absence of my company. I had to figure out a way to be both employee and mother, half here and half there, focused on the job and always thinking of her. But how? How was I expected to function and be of purpose when I had just kissed my newly-found purpose in life good-bye and left her to eat cereal and watch Curious George with her cousin? I really didn't know.

Tasks and time.

Turns out, by the end of my first week back at work, I had come to the conclusion that the anticipation of the return to work had been entirely more brutal than the actual return. Many of my fears (her survival, my survival, Katie's survival) had been put to rest and we had all made it through the week relatively unscathed. Emotionally, there had been new bridges and barriers to breach. I hadn't expected I would sustain such deep pangs of missing such a small baby. I also hadn't anticipated the amount of joy I would feel when I walked through the door after an entire day of *being* missed. Both were steadily showing to be worthwhile.

Tasks at work began to generate more of my focus throughout the days ahead. I didn't have a very difficult job but it did take great organization, and that demanded my attention whether I wanted it to or not. No matter how much I resisted, my thoughts started to squeeze out concerns for my child (concerns that I had no control over anyway) and began to familiarize themselves with the routine of my work to which I had been accustomed prior to my leave.

Within a few weeks, no one was stopping me in the halls and asking about my baby anymore. I didn't need to keep a stash of Kleenex in my pocket just in case I got misty glancing at the photos on my desk. I stopped calling over the lunch hour to check in and see if she was predictably happy and well. I didn't like it any more than that awful first day, but simple routine had replaced the anxiety of my resistance. Although some days my acceptance of the situation probably resembled a lack of motivation to change the situation, I knew that deep down I was at my best to live in the current state we were managing at the moment and search for gratitude within the present.

I had been extraordinarily blessed. Not only did I have a healthy baby but I had a good job. That was more than anyone could have hoped for in this life, really. Again, it was the struggle within *myself* that was telling me I should be deserving of more, of better, of different. I had good motives. My discontent was strictly coming from what I deemed best for my daughter. But did that justify it?

23

Making the Most of a Messy Life

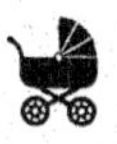

Complaining about life is normal. Everyone does it. Everywhere. Often. Sometimes complaining can motivate us to do more, be better, grow deeper, or endure longer.

Complaining, however, is one of those toxic, unseen, totally-acceptable diseases that most of us have. If you don't have it, you definitely know someone who does. We've all been around someone who was a chronic complainer, and honestly, I can't think of anything more wearing or futile. If complaining isn't the core symptom of selfishness, it is certainly its sister.

I was becoming dangerously close to becoming a master complainer. I was constantly catching myself on the verge of a complete and utter tantrum. And I knew it was wrong.

I don't like this project at work. I don't get along with my co-worker. I didn't get credit for that idea at the meeting. I didn't get to eat lunch with my friends. I didn't get to kiss Matilda good-bye because she was still asleep when I left for work. I didn't get to see her clap her hands at the TV. I didn't get to rock her to sleep for her nap. I didn't get to be there when she woke up. I didn't get to relax when I got home. I didn't get to catch up with my husband. I didn't have time to do the laundry. I didn't get to bed on time. I didn't get a full night's sleep.

It was all just too much. I couldn't live in a state of didn'ts or don'ts. My brain couldn't contain the amount of discontent my heart seemed to churn out each day. If I knew how truly blessed I really was, how come I didn't *feel* that way?

I wanted things to change, but I could only change myself. This is a common problem for the complainer, the avid, unwilling-to-budge, complainer. I felt so justified in wanting my circumstances to change that I hadn't ever taken the time to view them otherwise. The lesson remained the same—more Jesus, less me. Replace my natural instinct with the greater ambition. Close the window on my temporary problems and gain perspective of the grand scheme.

Stress has the tendency to limit your ability to appreciate the present. When I'm sitting in a state of calm and assurance, I can easily point out all the blessings and miracles around me that make me smile throughout the day. But when I feel pulled in a million directions and my attention becomes divided between all the little tasks that have yet to be done, I find myself looking at the clock, the to-do list, and the calendar instead of looking at what's right in front of my face.

PRAISE AND POOPY DIAPERS

When I look up the word *complain* in my thesaurus the first antonym listed is *praise*. Interesting. Sometimes, when you're trying hard to change habits, the first step can be as simple as a word search. The opposite of complaining is praising. Praising! Think about that. It's not keep your mouth shut or vent to your mother instead of your husband or even pray about it. Nope. It's praise.

Then I looked up the definition of the word *praise*, and this is what I found:

> **Praise** (noun)
>
> 1. words that express great approval or admiration, for example, for somebody's ability or achievements or for something's good qualities
>
> 2. worship and thanks to God or a deity (often used in the plural)
>
> (verb)

1. to express great approval or admiration, for example, for somebody's ability or achievements or for something's good qualities
2. to give worship and thanks to God or a deity

(Encarta® World English Dictionary © 1999 Microsoft Corporation. All rights reserved. Developed for Microsoft by Bloomsbury Publishing Plc.)

Reread that definition and just soak in these words: *approval, admiration, ability, achievements, good qualities, worship, thanks to God.*

I had to get out of my complaining rut if I was going to survive this new schedule and thrive at being a mother, if I wanted to love my husband and remain employed. I had to stop, drop, and roll out some serious praise.

Lucky for us, there is really no wrong way to praise God. If you're ever at a loss, the Bible is chock-full of amazing examples (start with the book of Psalms and go from there.) Singing, dancing, simply speaking aloud your thanks to the Lord are all amazing ways to focus your praise on Him and away from distress. Isn't it awesome that all the ways in which we can praise Jesus happen to also be intrinsically mood-lifting? When is the last time you sang a praise song and ended it in a foul mood? Or were grumpy after dancing? Or felt worse after giving thanks?

Praise is a game-changer. It is essential to gratitude. It is imperative for joy. And it is the best defense against unreasonable grouchiness that I know of!

PRAISE AMIDST THE MESS

I think there is a difference between praising God and just counting your blessings. Sometimes I can get in a prayer rut of thanking God for the same things over and over again. It's nearly superstitious, like if I forget to mention that I'm thankful for my health then I'm bound to get sick, or if I skip a day without being grateful for food, work, or money all of a sudden it will disappear.

But that's not how God works. He doesn't bless us according to what we do. He doesn't count how many times we say thank you and then check it off His list when we fulfill the quota. Thank goodness, this isn't how it works!

Instead, God chooses and allows blessings in our lives *in spite* of who we are and what we do. All good things come from God alone. All. It isn't because of our praise and our thanksgiving that He blesses us; it's because He blesses us that we are so incredibly, inevitably motivated to praise Him. When we complain, when we choose to focus on what we would rather have or do or when we decide that our God isn't fulfilling our needs (that *is* what complaining is when it comes down to it, now isn't it?) then we completely lose sight of all He has done for us.

WHEN YOUR ATTITUDE STINKS MORE THAN THE DIAPERS

When life is most messed, it isn't less blessed. And, believe me, parenting comes with a lot of messes! One of these moments sticks out in my mind, the day of the big blow-out. Now it's no mystery that babies come with stinky diapers. It's all part of the deal. But rarely do you know what a true blow out is until you have your own child and are the one solely responsible for clean up duty.

I had just taken Matilda on an outing when on our way back I could hear her filling up her diaper from the back seat of the car. Oh man, this was about to get real. I got her out of her car seat, took her into the house, and immediately knew I was in trouble. Sparing you the details (hey, you might be reading this on a lunch break after all) I skipped the changing table altogether and headed straight into our bathroom, starting the tub running.

I looked at this sad, squirming, stinky baby. She was covered in yuck. The onesie was beyond salvageable. Her pants were goners. I literally decided to get a small pair of scissors and cut the outfit off of the poor child to avoid further destruction! This, my friends, was a messy moment.

I was beyond grossed out, frustrated, and ready to start babbling complaints at how hard my life was, when suddenly I stared into the eyes of this silly little human covered in yuck. *My* silly little human. My messy life, stinky and ridiculous. And I burst into laughter instead of tears. Suddenly I was caught in a moment of praise instead of complaint.

Despite what we think or feel, we're all constantly living in a state of messing and blessing. Some seasons of our lives may be more difficult than others; some may not have much explanation; some may even run rampant with pain and sorrow. But our God is unchanging and ever giving. The world is unfair, but God is just. That is the truth.

So when I say we are motivated because He's blessed us, and you're sitting there thinking, "Maybe He's blessed you, but He didn't bless me!" You are dead wrong.

Boom! Did you shut the book on me? Wait! Stay with me here, and I promise not to judge you.

Jesus was God's ultimate blessing to us, all of us. Jesus is all we need. Jesus is everything. Jesus is enough. Jesus warrants infinite praise.

Case closed. Why, when we hear the word *blessing* do we so often jump to the idea of health and wealth? Why do I always start picturing all the things in my life I don't have? Why do I start praying as if I'm reading a revised copy of next year's Christmas list?

"Okay, Lord, I would like a bigger apartment and a car that doesn't squeal. I could use some nicer clothes that fit better, and it sure would be handy to get some new curtains for the living room. If you could throw in some new dining furniture, I could probably work on reading my Bible more often. Have we got ourselves a deal? Amen."

Yikes.

The big secret is—Jesus. Praising Jesus is the natural response to having a relationship with Him. It's not an obligation or a chore or a bummer in the middle of my day. It is a choice. It does take time. It does take energy, focus, and effort, just like any other relationship.

Now don't start feeling all guilty on me because you

haven't stopped to thank God for something. Just talk to Him about it. Get real and honest with God (helpful hint: He already knows everything anyway.) Soon enough, when you least expect it and maybe when you feel all gross and emotional and teary and messy from having bared your yucky soul, you will praise Him.

Praise is the opposite of complaining; being quiet is not. Praise. God doesn't want you to keep it all inside and have nowhere to put it. He doesn't want us marinating in toxic thoughts of waste that eat at us with no resolution. He is the only resolution, no matter how small or insanely large the complaint might be.

24

Why Superwoman Would Have Made a Great Working Mother

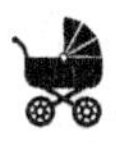

It turns out God became my ultimate de-stressor. Turning away from complaining and toward praise and thanksgiving (don't save it just for the month of November!) was slowly digging me out of my pessimistic rut. It didn't change my circumstances. It changed everything else, which was far more powerful.

My routine became just that—routine—and soon enough I was chugging along habit-by-habit as if having a baby had only been a hiccup in the course of my otherwise-perfectly scheduled life. Every morning, I was up and dressed by 7 a.m. I'd feed, change, and dress the baby by 7:30 a.m. and get her set up in her high chair with some sort of breakfast gruel by the time Katie and Sofie showed up to take over. Josh and I would carpool in to work, kiss good-bye at the lobby, and go our separate ways to our separate departments, travel mugs brimming with coffee to get us through the morning. Routine.

I was learning to be content where I was. I was trying to make the best of a pretty good situation, which should have been a lot easier than it seemed at the time. I fell into a rhythm of knowing who would want to hear about Matilda's latest-and-greatest accomplishments ("She blew a kiss this morning! It nearly melted my heart!") and who couldn't care less. I felt new boundaries around the workplace that I hadn't felt prior to having my baby. Some people seemed to feel my pain with one look, knowing in a single glance I must have been up all night with the baby and offering a slight tilt of the head with a smile that told me they'd been there before. Other people—kid-free, heartless robots let's call them—blatantly rolled their eyes any time baby talk came up or I had anything to say that somehow revolved around the notion that I had a baby to take into consideration.

Some people will never understand your priorities, no matter how hard you try. Sometimes these same people are even parents themselves, and it can become infuriating to wonder how they ever survived entrance into parenthood without ample support or similar compassion. Who knows?

ALL HANDS TO THE PUMPS

But there was something in this new routine of mine that I never quite adjusted to—breastfeeding. I was determined to keep breastfeeding while returning to work. I knew it wouldn't be easy, but frankly, that's about all I knew about it.

A few weeks before returning to work, I had tried to schedule the baby's feedings rather than just nurse her on demand. When your baby is screaming and your breasts are filling up like water balloons, you throw your schedule out the window and nurse your baby as soon as possible. That being said, I wasn't very conditioned by the time I made my transition back into the working world.

My body felt like a ticking time bomb. I think I wore two sets of nursing pads and brought an extra sweater that whole first week back at work "just in case" my milk went haywire all over my wardrobe. As much as you read and learn through books, there is pretty much no preparing you for the let down feeling when your milk fills up your breasts. It's painful and weird and sort of tingly in a super uncomfortable way, and even though absolutely no one will notice it's happening, you get the sensation that everyone is looking at your giant melon-boobs that feel like they are going to burst. Whoa, mama. It's crazy.

Needless to say, if I was going to continue to feed my baby breast milk, it was imperative that I pump during the day and store up what she would eat while I was at work. But when? When was I supposed to just politely excuse myself and be gone for half an hour and return with a lunch bag of milk to store in the employees' break-room fridge? How exactly was I going to discreetly transport my giant electric pump in and out of a private spot without someone wondering what the heck was up?

I had a lot of questions before jumping into this new world of milk provision. It was intimidating. It was scary. And I wondered the whole time how in the world every working, breastfeeding, mother seems to somehow figure all this out and glide through her day as if it was something covered the first day of orientation on the job. Say, what?

Luckily, I knew some women who had walked this road before me. I was still intimidated, but I found some friendly faces that were able to point me in the right direction (and I took notes!) I boldly decided it was worth the risk of trying it out for myself. There was only one teensy catch—I worked almost exclusively with men!

At first, this made me incredibly uncomfortable. I envisioned nightmares of leaking through my blouse during important meetings or having to excuse myself and being asked why and I would have to politely explain that I needed to pump my breast milk, thank you very much. But then I realized how insanely embarrassed that would most likely make *them*—far more embarrassed than I would probably ever be (after all, it's not my fault I'm trying to sustain a life back home!) and I figured this whole pumping gig could nearly be my get-out-of-jail-free card if I ever needed or wanted a reason to promptly excuse myself. Nice. It was that whole give-the-old-gym-teacher-a-sad-face-and-they-will-let-you-sit-out-of-running-that-day-because-it's-too-awkward-a-situation-to-ask-you-directly-why sort of understanding that just might come in handy if need be.

I'm glad to say I never had to escape work to go pump

unexpectedly. But it was still nice to know I had the embarrassment-upper-hand if it ever came down to it. Now if I could just figure out the darn schedule.

It was a few weeks of awkward excuses before my body adjusted to a pattern. Milk production is a super-weird concept and entirely individual depending on each mother's and baby's needs. I know women with enormous breasts who barely produce any milk and always struggle to feed enough. I know women with tiny breasts who could feed a small village for a year. There doesn't seem to be much rhyme or reason for what we're doled out, but for myself I was blessed with the bosoms of a dairy cow. In other words, I had no problem always producing plenty (or more) than what my baby needed. This was wonderful, but it also meant that it took a little more time for my body to decide when to and when not to let down and have milk ready. This was especially frustrating since I was still nursing my baby on-demand when I was at home.

Finally, after a couple months of lugging my electric pump wherever I went, I was able to settle into a pattern of pumping over my lunch break only. Whew!

Fortunately, some brilliant woman-engineer somewhere designed the modern electric pump to resemble a sort of leather messenger bag. I would fit any extra components in my purse, along with whatever novel I was currently reading, and I would promptly leave my cubicle as soon as I was able to break for lunch.

SECRET AGENT MAMA: BOND. JANE BOND. BREAST-FEEDING 007

Here's the main thing I discovered when talking to all those working moms who dealt with this before me: the breastfeeding working mother has to become a secret agent.

I promise, if you don't think you know or see any breastfeeding women, you do. It's just that they fly totally under the radar until you are in the club.

It must be one of those things you just never see because you never think about it until you have to. Because I found out there was an entirely secret room—they called this magical land the "nursing lounge"—where you could go and pump in private, tucked away from the rest of civilization. It had an entry code on the power-locked door and everything, totally James-Bond style. But unfortunately, it was in another building a decent walk away from the building where I worked.

The clock would strike noon, and I would grab my gear and dart through the lobby on my mission. I only took thirty minutes for lunch most days, so in order to get there, pump, eat lunch, and run I really had to book.

Working wardrobes are not conducive to this lifestyle. Never have I found a good zip-up-the-back dress that had a tag on it reading "Great for the working mom who breast pumps!" Never. As soon as I entered my code and walked into the nursing lounge (okay, even though it was called the nursing lounge, it was truly more like a nursing closet—a tiny room with a chair, sink, lamp, and one plug-in ready, no waiting) I would lock the door and quickly change like Superman in a phone booth (which was really ironic since the room was about as big as a phone booth.)

Flash! *Kapow*! I could assemble that sucker (no pun intended) in about seven seconds flat. I got so good that I could pump both breasts, eat a peanut-butter-and-jelly sandwich, and read *Twilight* all at the same time (and not spill a drop!) I would pack up, do my superhero-quick change one more time, and—*Voila!*—I walked the sidewalks as a normal human being once more, no one the wiser as to how I'd spent the last half hour.

It sounds silly, but it was a huge component to my day. No one in my whole department knew exactly where I was or what I was doing for that thirty-minute period. I mean, I might as well have been out in a cape fighting crime, right? Maybe not. I certainly felt like a secret agent sneaking in and out of coded doors, undressing and redressing quick as a flash and assembling gear for which the average person would have questioned its use.

It was a far cry from the lunch break I took prior to motherhood. Back in those days, lunchtime was a chorus of camaraderie. Josh had several coworkers in his department who had become our closest friends, and I would always meet them at the on-campus dining spot where we would nibble our food and gnaw on the news of the day. Often, we'd have to push two or three tables together just to accommodate everyone. It wasn't just a break from the workday; it was friendship! On the days when not everyone could meet up, Josh and I could still make a lunch date out of the time and truly take advantage of working in the same location.

I knew when I came back to work that I would miss those times, especially because I knew what I was missing. I mean, it isn't like those times stopped just because I wasn't there. It was more like I knew that just yards away were tables where my friends were getting together and gabbing over tuna sandwiches about how ghastly-awful their morning workday had been. If you've ever worked a day in your life, you understand how necessary it can be to get a little validation in the middle of the day to keep you motivated.

Still, I knew I was choosing what I wanted. I deeply valued nursing my baby and keeping her on breast milk for as long as I could sustain it. If that meant locking myself in a closet and chewing p-b-and-j sandwiches over the whirring sound of an electric pump, well, so be it.

A few resentful and intimidating days into this routine, I discovered I liked it. No, I loved it. This little nursing closet was more than just a convenient resource for me. It was my haven.

Listen to that! Did you hear it? *Vrrrrrrrrrrr*. Silence. All I could hear was the steady rhythm of the pump, and that was it. It was startling how calming it was when I stopped to notice it. I bet somebody could have hypnotized me right then and there (of course, they would have had to know the code to get in.)

Day after day, I found myself rushing to get to my little closet of comfort, not just because I had 8 ounces of milk to pump in twenty minutes flat, but also because I needed the mental rest away from the outside world. This time was *mine*. Alone. Away. All mine. In the midst of needs from the baby, the coworker, the husband, the boss, and the rest of the world,

I really started to crave that moment of silence. And a moment was all it took to hit my reset button, recharge my attitude and energy, and be able to tackle the rest of the day with worthwhile intention.

This revelation of needing a moment to myself was going to serve me well in the long run of parenthood. I had always heard from other mothers about getting "me time," and honestly, I usually equated that with weakness. But when it became organically forced upon me out of sheer schedule and necessity, I had no choice but to stop long enough to appreciate it and to start seeing the amazing value it could extend into the rest of my day/life.

After several months, I began to find myself with leftover minutes in the lunch break. Now, you tell me, what's a tired girl to do with a quiet room, a chair, and extra minutes to spare?

I napped in that nursing closet more than I ever did in my own bed at home—I guarantee it. As my baby became less dependent on breast milk, the less I had to pump and the less time it took up in my day. By several months in, I would only spend the first few minutes pumping. Then I would set an alarm on my phone, turn out the light, and lay my head back (or very uncomfortably curl up) on the chair. Night, night!

I'll admit it—for the first few months after Matilda stopped nursing altogether, I continued my routine of going to that nursing closet for the sole purpose of catching a few Zs in the middle of the day. The nursing closet officially became my private napping closet for many weeks until I started to feel guilty when I found out someone else—an actual nursing mother—needed to book the room. Granted, by this time I had another excuse for my extreme fatigue as I was already pregnant with my second child, but let's save that story for another book, another time.

25

Motherhood: The Ultimate Job

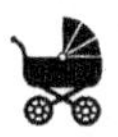

I never loved work. Despite my driven nature, I have never been one of those "career women" who wanted to sport a power suit and carry a Burberry briefcase and make major decisions that other men in suits would smugly nod at. I've pretty much always looked at work as a means to an end (a necessary paycheck) and tried my best to figure out a job that utilized my gifts while meeting my needs at the same time. Even though I knew I would have to continue working once the baby arrived, I never thought my attitude towards work would change after returning. But it did.

I was no longer just meeting my needs. I was no longer just getting a paycheck. I was partnering up with my husband to provide a lifestyle I had always dreamed of. I was eagerly working toward a new goal—staying home for good. I didn't know how or when, but going back to work and leaving my baby behind had sealed the deal for me in knowing what career choice I needed to make, and everything else up until then was just going to be practice toward that goal. I wanted to be a stay-at-home mom for sure.

It was difficult and emotionally taxing to get up and go to

work with this new goal in my heart. I had known it in my head all along, but it took actually going back to work to confirm the decision in my heart. Even though I had never wanted to leave my baby at home, I suppose I'd had thoughts like "Would I wonder what it was like to go back to work if I never had the chance?" I'm glad I experienced the painful and awkward entry back into the workforce, if for no other reason than to gain a deep appreciation for the moms who have to do it every day and for the joy of knowing what it is to be missed by your child.

I didn't just want my time at work to pass without my taking advantage of it, either. I don't mean the naps in the nursing closet (though that was a perk!) but I'm talking about the little (and mostly overlooked) joys that work can bring to your day and throughout your life.

Working in an office definitely taught me many things: time management, schedule keeping, how to prioritize and work efficiently under pressure, and how to focus on one task at a time. I began to look at my job as a stepping-stone to my future goal. How could my job strengths transition into effective motherhood?

THERE'S NO SUCH THING AS A NONWORKING MOTHER

I had found a new praise-centric mindset being able to look at this daily work as a practice field for honing the skills I would need to someday run my own household. I'm not saying I was going to start charting out laundry duties or setting Google calendars for taking out the trash, but I definitely began to see how God was going to utilize my skills in the home just as much (or more) as He had in my work life.

As much as I couldn't leave my new mothering lifestyle on the doorstep of my apartment when I went to work, I couldn't just turn off my time-management skills when I clocked out. As simple as it sounds, I took myself wherever I went. And this was a new revelation for me. Just as motherhood was becoming ingrained in my very being, the 30-some-odd jobs I had worked throughout my history of employment had been coming to fruition for their ultimate cause—shaping me into the person I was supposed to be, the person I was.

It is strange how we all think we know what we need when truly, if I'm being completely honest, my list of needs is nothing more than wants I believe I deserve. This can be a dangerous place from which to approach the throne of grace. Again, it made me re-evaluate how I was praying, how I was speaking to my Creator, and how I began asking Him for His will instead of my own. It seems fundamental to a relationship with Jesus but something I so easily forget—what God wants for us is always going to be greater than what we think we need.

Maybe you don't have to go back to work after your baby is born. Maybe you already know your life's dream is going to be fulfilled by staying home. Or maybe you are choosing to return to work because you want to rather than need to. Regardless of the circumstance, God is using your lifestyle in your mothering and your mothering in your lifestyle. There's no reversing its effects, either.

I was a working mother. I was a mother, working. I was a work in progress employed by God for more than a job—I had found my true vocation.

26

Planet Parenthood

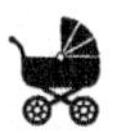

When I became a mother, I expected myself to change. I knew something extraordinary was happening to my body, entering my life, and changing the world as I knew it for the rest of my time here on Earth. I knew I would look in the mirror and see someone new—a mother, whatever that may mean—someone exclusively needed by someone else, someone trying to unconditionally love a new little being. I knew I would be different *to me.*

But I don't think I realized that when I became a mother I would also become someone entirely new *to other people* as well. This thought never really occurred to me, as simple and fundamental as it may sound.

We were the first of the majority of our friends to have a baby, pioneers, if you will. So it seemed natural to us that our life would pretty much carry on as usual, just with a baby in tow. I mean, sure, we knew there would be less sleep, more crying, and definitely a need for some new boundaries, but without a little person actually here in real life it was difficult to understand what this might entail prior to the baby's arrival.

This is similar to when we (like many couples) thought

before getting married that marriage would be just like dating except for the fact that we got to have sex whenever we wanted and hang our clothes in the same closet.

And that is similar to the expectation I had before going away (several states away, mind you) to college, thinking college was a four-year camp away from home where you finally got to stay up late and eat whatever you want whenever you want to.

Where the heck do we come up with these dreamy ideas? Maybe I've watched too many movies. As you can guess, none of these expectations were met. Instead, one by one, like crazy-life dominos they toppled over with a giant crash, each predictable and yet still a shocking surprise to me all the same.

No doubt, most life-changing events are simply that—life-changing. If they met our expectations as we thought they would, we'd most likely just go on our happy-go-lucky way as if nothing new had ever taken place. Where's the excitement in that?

SEEING THE WORLD THROUGH THE EYES OF A PARENT

Here I was, a newly-changed person now called "Mom" and all of a sudden I felt like every person I'd ever known was staring at me cockeyed and questioning whom I had become. The craziest thing about it all was that I totally didn't care. From the second somebody walked in the door I was all about baby this, baby that, baby, baby, baby. It sounds cliché, but I can't remember asking anybody anything about their life within the first six weeks of having a baby. I can't tell you who did what or why, not even about my dearest friends! But I can tell you the exact day I first saw my baby smile, and I can tell you about our first outing with her (from what she wore to what we ate at brunch) and I can perfectly picture the first time I heard her giggle. The point is that my priorities had changed forever. Forever! Not just for those first six weeks but for the rest of my life.

Was it fair? No. Was it expected? No. Did it matter? Yes.

Totally, it mattered. Those first few months were such a daze that I basically wore baby goggles and saw everything from an entirely new world view with my baby as the center of my universe. Everything else was just too challenging or too boring to deal with at the moment. Everything else could wait. At least, it seemed that way.

To a point, this is good and healthy. But of course no one can survive without the help of others, so it's good to remember that your friends *are* indeed important. After all, they threw you that lovely baby shower, they baked you that casserole, and they bought you that ugly onesie they really hope you put your baby in very soon.

GET YOUR BABY GOGGLES READY

Baby goggles are pretty much inevitable. You went through a life-changing experience, and though you might be the better for it, you can't deny its effect on your daily life. Your life is never going to be the same and neither are your friendships. The sooner you learn this and accept it, the easier and more fulfilling it will all become.

Baby goggles happen for three reasons:

1. You don't have the luxury of time.
2. You don't have the luxury of sleep.
3. You don't have the luxury of perpetual concern.

You've just landed on a new planet, planet Parenthood, and this world is entirely baby-centric. You, your time, your energy, your focus, your worry, your patience, your values, are now entirely wrapped around the obstacle and privilege now known as your child. It may sound like a joke, like something you read in a baby shower card from Hallmark, but the truth is as soon as you set eyes on your baby, you'd willingly hand over all your possessions simply to hold her, be with her, care for her. This is that new-found love you've been waiting for, that love only other parents have told you about. That love you never knew you always wanted to feel but couldn't ever put into words. The love of having a child.

It's beautiful. It's nearly perfect. It's pretty much as close as we can get to experiencing the kind of love God has for us.

The only difference is that God doesn't want to throw a baby bottle through the window at 3 a.m. when His child won't stop crying, and we do. (Can I get an *Amen*?)

Nevertheless, we return to our child again and again, giving up ourselves, our sleep, our time, so that we can be there for her whenever she needs us. This, truly, is the miracle that is parenthood. This is why having a baby is the perfect recipe for seeking God, because the truth is children can wear on you so deeply that you are stripped of everything else and have nowhere else to turn. I don't know where I would be, let alone where my child would be, if I didn't have prayer to turn to in the middle of all the joyous wonder that is this crazy, selfless journey.

HALF-PAST POOP AND TWENTY MINUTES TILL EAT

The first thing baby goggles strip you of is time. Your time. This happens extraordinarily in a variety of ways. Time warps when you are awakened at intervals of two to three hours. You don't recognize the numbers on the clock because they don't have the words *eat* or *poop* next to them, and those are the only real times you keep track of. You can't remember the day of the week because there is no longer a weekend off work to look forward to. Time exists as "how long until I get to sleep again?" and that's all.

There is no more being lazy. There is no more "killing time." There is only soaking up the splendor, enjoying the moment, or sleeping, and in between all of that you are just struggling to keep your baby happy.

Baby goggles are even less concerned with your need for sleep than they are for time. It's true that some people have sweetly-sleeping babies. I've heard legends about babies who come home from the hospital, sleep in their crib on the first try or sleep through the night from the get-go. I've come to realize that I either have to hate these parents or simply believe them to be untrue tellers of baby lore, so I prefer the latter.

My baby was not of the sleeping kind. I was convinced

from the beginning that she either hated me or hated sleep. Of course I went with the theory that she hated sleep and therefore loved me so entirely that she simply couldn't stand the thought of departing my presence, so she forced herself to stay awake out of sheer delight in being with me. This thought, however, still didn't provide me the deep rest my body longed for. The long *eight months* of her waking every *two hours* certainly took its toll on my mind, my work, my patience, and my coffee intake.

Sleep was rough in our house. There is only so much a friend can do for you when all you have to say is "I'm sorry. I'm so tired." Therefore, it took its toll on friendships too. It's one thing to sit and tell someone how tired you are, but no one really gets it unless they are living it too (think back to college all-nighters and you'll get an idea of what I'm talking about.)

The final thing baby goggles strip you of is the luxury of perpetual concern. This may sound brutal, but after you have a baby most of the other drama surrounding your friends just loses its luster. It's really hard to care about some of their problems when you are suddenly placed in charge of a tiny, all-new human being who relies on you entirely for her survival. You don't have the luxury of caring about your friend not getting a text back from the cute boy she's interested in. You don't have the fortitude to listen to how your friend is still looking for a new apartment near the beach. You simply don't care whether your friend got looked over again for the promotion they were hoping for.

Baby goggles are just one of those things you are sure will never happen to you when you have kids, but it does. And the thing is, you can't help it. And the *real* thing is, you wouldn't want it any other way. You and your friends will most likely end up walking away from each other thinking the exact same thing: "They just don't understand!"

27

Now You Know Who Your True Friends Really Are

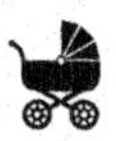

Friendships are strange. They are wonderful and necessary and entirely essential to building community and, therefore, a successfully happy life on this earth. There are all kinds of friendships—from the nice acquaintance at work to the friend who makes you laugh until you snort.

I love friends. I couldn't make it through this life without the people who love and support my family and me. But of all the friends in all the world who have blessed my life, there is only one kind of friend that stands out above the rest—the friend without expectation.

I never knew this even existed prior to becoming a parent, but I will never take it for granted now that I know what it means. The friend without expectation is the first true friend you need after having a baby. Maybe you already know who this is. Maybe you will be right! Chances are you won't really know who this person is until they've proven to you how much you need them. And if you're lucky, maybe you will have an entire community without expectation that can support you in the early days.

The essential thing to remember about a friend without expectation is that they don't ever question your baby goggles. In fact, they never resent you for wearing them in the first place and usually help you put them on. They might even ask if you have an extra pair around so they can pretend to have baby goggles too!

A true friend is going to be baby-centric about your baby too. They're going to be so overjoyed for you, so eager to learn more about your life, so excited to be part of this life-changing event that your complete lack of interest in their life is going to seemingly go unnoticed for the first several visits from this friend. You need this friend. Just don't take them for granted.

This friend totally gets that you mean them no disregard by completely disregarding them. They understand that you mean no disinterest by totally ignoring them. And they absolutely would be offended if you *didn't* tend to your child as soon as she needed you, even if they were in the middle of a grand story about their own life.

FRIENDS NEED FRIENDS TOO

But here's the thing about this magical friend without expectation—they only last for a very short window of time. After all, they're human too, and you've been in baby la-la-land for a while now. All that time, they're storing up gobs and gobs of stories to vent on you when that seemingly-appropriate time presents itself, and they're seriously beginning to wonder when that time might be (or if that time might ever be!)

Don't take this friend for granted. Cherish the sacred time with your new baby, yes. Tend to your challenging, all-demanding, newly-found parenthood, yes. But, understand that you are only excused from reality a short while before your true and caring friends start to wonder if they've been forever replaced by a cute bundle of cries that demands your every focus.

Friends are part of life's joys and blessings. I have some friends who continue to amaze me and listen to me and go far above and beyond to help me through life's challenges. These friends *want* to be there for me and count it a privilege to engage in my life. Sometimes this kind of love is hard to accept. Sometimes it's hard to understand why someone would actually choose to come over and fold laundry for me while I take a nap or nurse the baby. Sometimes it's beyond all my reason to grasp how I could possibly ever give back to them in the way they give to me, which is exactly what makes them necessary to my life and exactly what makes them a friend *without* expectation.

But there comes a time shortly following the birth when you need to start engaging back into the friendships around you. Your nearest and dearest may extend you extra grace for a proper adjustment period, but don't push it. Keep your boundaries, pace yourself, do the best you can, and when in doubt, thank them for just being around.

Somewhere between the time of mastering breastfeeding and returning to your prepregnancy jeans (hopefully sooner than later!) you should begin splitting your attention. It's time to remove the baby goggles. It's time to look up and ask questions about others' lives. It's time to return the grace that was extended to you. And for heaven's sake, wash and return those casserole pans before you forget who they belong to!

28

Back to the Future

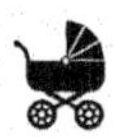

Here's the truth. This will be no fun and it will feel a little bit sad and pitiful for you. You may want to bite your spoiled tongue before you roll your eyes one more time. You are under the influence of what I call "the unicorn effect."

When you are pregnant, a whole new world opens up for you. Certainly, this is a scary world, a realm of new worries and anxieties beyond your wildest imagination. You've been getting bumped up a space in line for the women's restroom, getting asked if you need anything on an hourly-ish basis, having doors opened for you, or getting rides to places you used to walk to.

THE UNICORN EFFECT

When you're pregnant, people go out of their way for you. They stare at you in wonder and sympathy. As a good friend of mine (who was great with child at the time she said this) joked that people gawk as if you are "a magical unicorn." The unicorn effect, if you will. Pregnancy ushers in a whole host of amazing endeavors, but one great perk is the fact that for nine-ish months of your life you become a celebrity of sorts. You really have no say over it. There's nothing you can do to stop it. People simply want to offer you a helpful hand, and it's probably somewhere deeply rooted in the fact that we can never fully repay our own mother for the nine months she endured toting us around in her magical womb.

Obviously, being pregnant is not without its discomforts, but I would be remiss not to mention the benefits the unicorn effect has on the expectant mother's life. It's wonderful. It's special. It's sacred. And then . . . it's gone.

FROM UNICORN TO BROODMARE

It might sound superficial or even selfish, but the truth is that when that baby pops out of you, you can no longer play the I-am-sorry-I-can't-do-such-and-such-because-I'm-so-gosh-darn-pregnant card. And the but-I-just-had-a-baby-I'm-not feeling-up-to-it card expires shortly after. Months and months of people caring for you, asking how you are feeling, reaching out to meet your needs and accommodating your every comfort . . . *BAM*. Done. You immediately fall back into the shuffle of the masses, regular joes and total suckers, having to fend for yourself again. You've gone from magical unicorn to boring broodmare all in one night. Shucks. That stinks.

Of course, you are so glad to get that baby out of you. As pleasant and wonderful as pregnancy is, I can still recall the final weeks of utter discomfort taking their toll on my body and my life. Definitely, by the end of my pregnancy the last thing I wanted was to remain that way forever. But there is something confusing and shocking about losing that unicorn effect. Suddenly you've returned to your normal skin (albeit a little stretched out and forever changed in your heart and soul by parenthood) and people don't look at you as if something surreal and supernatural just happened to you. But *it did*!

It can be disconcerting, to say the least. One moment people were opening doors for you and smiling at your growing belly, and the next week you're exhausted, covered in poop and breast milk, and everyone just wants to hold the baby while you're left with a jelly belly you were promised by

Glamour magazine should be whittled down to normal by now (at least, that's what happened to Heidi Klum, right?) It can all just seem entirely unfair.

I loved my new baby. LOVED. Could not have been more thrilled about her arrival. But, amidst all the excitement and enthusiasm and complete and utter joy that surrounded her arrival, suddenly I was lost among the aftermath that paved the way for her perfect entrance. And I missed the attention. I missed my paparazzi, the unicorn onlookers, that is. I missed my celebrity status.

The last thing I wanted to do was be jealous of my new baby. Scratch that—the last thing I wanted to do was resent my new baby. I mean, she's a baby! That's just preposterous. Besides, I was too tired and too preoccupied in those first few weeks to even recognize that I felt a void when my paparazzi left. I was too distracted with the pain of recovery and the insane new schedule to even think twice about why in the world I wanted to be asked more about how I was feeling, doing, or being.

It was super easy to chalk all my emotions up to postpartum, to recovery pain meds, or to lack of sleep. Besides, lots of people did ask me right after the birth how I was handling the recovery and brutal reality of motherhood as a first-timer, so it wasn't like I was completely disregarded when visitors would come by.

Still, as the weeks swiftly passed, fewer and fewer people acknowledged me in public. No glances, no helping hands of strangers, no unicorn gawkers at the ready for me to rely on to open doors for me and my new bulky stroller or let me cut in line for the handicap stall so I could nurse in the middle of a Target shopping trip. Turns out, while everyone loves a cute baby, people are not so keen on a cranky new mom with no patience. Go figure.

This kind of reality can feel harsh to a new mom who just needs a hug. I'm not sure there is much preparation you can do besides me sitting here trying to reset your expectations accordingly. I didn't even understand this was what I was feeling until months after getting over it and growing a bit thicker skin.

Crying spells at three in the morning have a tendency to develop this for you; it's amazing.

I will say this: I missed the wonder of pregnancy. I didn't even know I missed it, but when I realized it I had to take a moment and think about it. I had to stop and grieve the loss of having her inside my body, all the while rejoicing in the incomparable miracle it was to hold her on the outside. It was a new phase, this holding-a-perfect-baby-who-was-mine phase of life, and yet it left in its quake an empty womb that had worked incredibly hard to make a fine home for months and months.

Most friends mean well. Hardly anyone was actually bummed out that we were having a baby. At least to our faces, people were overjoyed and thoughtful and encouraging even though over half of them had no idea what they were really encouraging us about. Nevertheless, our announcement of the birth of our child was overwhelmingly met with congratulations and well wishes.

29

The Joys and Jealousies of Friends Without Kids

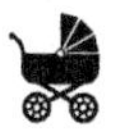

In the category of friendship, far from the end of the spectrum where the friend-without-expectation lies is the other side of friendship, the friends who will disappoint you. The friends who will drop you. The friends who will ultimately stop inviting you to things simply based on the fact that you have a kid now and they're not sure how "all that" fits into their footloose-and-fancy-free, perfectly-organized, spit-up-free, childless world. You know, where you used to live?

Aha, the nonparent friend. Don't get me wrong, some nonparent friends make for the absolute best allies on the planet. In fact, the nonparent-but-hope-to-someday-be-a-parent friend is your only link to a sane world for a while when you are acclimating yourself back to reality once the baby is born. They will stare in awe of you, want to support you, and maybe even want to learn from you as they watch your every move in amazement as if you are the Jedi master of all parents. It will weird you out, but just go with it and enjoy it. You probably stared at someone like that at some point, and that's exactly how you got the idea to warm up the baby wipe in your hand before it touched the baby's bottom and scared her to death or how you came up with that lullaby you can't stop humming or where that notion settled in your brain that you should just keep the coffee pot on all day instead of reheating the same cup again and again.

Parenthood is nothing if it is not a training ground for someday-parents to reap from the lessons and trials of our daily life. Nonparents are always watching, taking notes, and absorbing our little tricks that get us from point A to point Sleep. Nonparents can be incredible company, so don't exclude them as an entirety when I move on to this next friend type.

Which leads me back to the not-so-sympathetic, childless friends that might drop you like a dirty beat on an Iggy Azalea track. *Boom.* Ouch.

GOOD-BYE, FAIR WEATHER FRIEND

It's going to happen. No new parent ever thinks it will happen to *them.* And no new parent wants it to happen to them. But somewhere, sometime, probably within the first year of your new baby's life, some friend will stop being your friend.

It's one of those unpredictable certainties of life, and I hate to be the one to break it to you. I can already tell you are shimmying through the Rolodex in your head trying to figure out A, who you hope it is or B, who you think it is. Let me stop you right there. You just won't know until it happens.

It was a slow discovery for us. Amidst the flurry of visitors right after Matilda's birth, everyone was so thoughtful and generous. Sure, So and So might not have come to visit right away, but he has that job that requires so much. Or yeah, that one couple couldn't make it to her dedication, but they live far enough away that it's understandable. And then . . . months have gone by. Maybe even a year. And all of a sudden, I had to look up on Facebook to see where to send a Christmas card to friends we used to see on a weekly basis before our baby was born.

I couldn't believe it. We had lost touch with *them*? Had this new bundle of joy become such an anchor in our lives that we were permanently tethered to shore while our friends drifted away? And then I would look down and see my baby smile, and the only thought that crossed my mind was this: *They really missed out.* The End.

I mean, wow. Sad. If our having a baby was reason enough to not invite us to a birthday party or a get-together, fine. But I'm not going to waste energy feeling guilty for moving forward with my life just because it might inconvenience someone else. The fact is that having a child means I'm not going to be there for a friend at some point in time when I *am* going to have to be there for my child. I can't be there for everybody all the time. I can be there for my child almost all the time, and that's about as good as I can imagine. So, friends wait. And real friends understand that.

I have some childless friends who love to travel. Not just travel like in-state or to-see-family sort of travel. No, I mean the real deal. Stamp-filled passports, robust backpacks, broken-in boots sort of traveling. Gutsy European-type explorers who somehow fit in wherever they go. These are the people you get jealous of when you don't hear from them for a month and suddenly you see their Twitter feed pop up in the middle of Switzerland, and all you can think is that the closest you've come to that life is reading J. R. R. Tolkien in eighth grade. (This revelation is always followed by many deep sighs and an urgent desire to re-watch *Lord of the Rings.*)

I remembered these friends telling me about how wonderfully unpredictable their lives were. I could see the enthusiasm and passion in their eyes as they spoke about how free they felt, just loving the sheer ability to disregard "daily life" and take off on an adventure all their own. It was romantic, it was inspiring, and it was limitless as long as children didn't interrupt their plans.

I remembered listening, seriously contemplating the depth of the life-altering decision I had made to have a child. I felt the weight of that burden sink onto my shoulders, the heavy expectation of forever bearing down on my heart as I envisioned a life of freedom slipping through my hands. And then, I looked down at my child—my tether—and all I wanted to do was tighten the grip and hang on for dear life.

RAISING A CHILD IS LIKE BEING A WORLD TRAVELER

Is my child going to keep me from experiencing some things in life? Sure, maybe. But my having her is also going to open up unbelievable corners of the universe that have never been seized. She is uncharted territory. She is a whole new land. She is an unpredictable, impossible adventure at her very core. What more is there to want to explore?

It was somewhere in this thought process that I realized I had made the right decision for myself. Perhaps my jet-setting friends would consider my joy a coping mechanism for coming to grips with what I was really giving up. But I don't think so. I chose parenthood, and it seems to have chosen me just the same. My journey was just beginning, and the map had no borders.

Deliberate. Scary. Breathtaking. Parenthood is the ultimate voyage, and in a short nine months I had gone from tourist to guide.

30

Parenthood: The Great Adventure

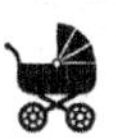

It's a little silly if I stop and think about it now, to consider my entire value system being adjusted, my priorities changed, my appreciation of what is truly important getting altered entirely, and to not think that my relationships would be affected. Crazyville. I didn't consider how my friendships would change after having a baby. I think I was too preoccupied with my husband, my waistline, and my registry at Target to look beyond what else needed my attention.

This is not to say that friendships don't come with a grace period when you get to steal the limelight for a bit. After all, when your best friend gets engaged, by all means you climb aboard her attention wagon and throw petals and parties in her honor. After you've had your baby and the next gal pal announces her expectancy, you graciously pass the torch (and your well-worn copy of *What to Expect When You're Expecting*) on to her so her belly can lead the parade for a while. There are just times in life when the unwritten rules of friendship take over, everyone bows accordingly, and you smile until it's your turn again.

As your world becomes smaller and smaller (think size-of-your-living-room kind of small) the rest of the planet is moving on without you. While you're trying to capture your baby's first rollover on your iPhone, you will have friends somewhere doing something super cool and fun and not kid-friendly at all. You'll see other people's status updates reminding you about these super cool and fun and not-kid-friendly-at-all activities. And you will miss them. You will miss your friends. And it will be too late.

And it will be worth it.

Maybe you used to go to clubs, throw darts at a bar, or hang out till 3 a.m. Maybe you used to play Yahtzee in your neighbor's basement and eat Rice Krispies Treats. Maybe you used to get up early and go running with your best friend or hit up a hot yoga class in the evenings. It doesn't really matter what kind of mischief you were into. Now your world has changed forever, and those days just aren't part of your life. And you know the strangest part about it all? Once you have a baby, you don't even really care.

I know; it's weird. You're scared part of you might die and you'll never get a chance to be that free bird who was going to go parasailing or send a drink to a stranger across a crowded room. Take a deep breath, and remember—your life's not over!

Just like you may have wondered the night before your wedding whether you would ever miss those crazy, dramatic dating days staying up all hours of the night pondering "the one," you knew as you walked down the aisle that your husband was the absolute, only soulmate for your forever. Right?

Well, in a way, becoming a parent is a similar feat. There's no turning back, and you wouldn't want it any other way. Nothing any friend ever says or does or posts on Facebook is going to make you want to take back having that perfect little human in your life. It may make you want to get a babysitter who is reliable and cheap, but that's about all.

Your new human is going to make you reevaluate everything in your life, and this includes the company you keep. Your friends are not truly your friends if they don't support your value system. If making your family a central priority in your life (including your energy, time, and money) isn't foremost in your value system, then you've read way too much of this book to care so little and I simply don't believe you. You care about your family. I can tell that much.

YOU NEED THOSE NONPARENT FRIENDS

You may lose touch with some friends for a while, but I encourage you to keep that bridge open as much as possible, no matter how far it may reach. After all, chances are pretty good that someday those crazy friends of yours just might get hitched or just might end up pregnant and just might ask you for some advice or hand-me-downs.

The best you can do for friends who drop you post-baby is to default to compassion. Empathize as much as you can, and vicariously live through their wild tales of freedom. Try to imagine how you might feel if you were they. Have you even asked them what's new in their life lately? Or are you too busy blabbing about missed naps and diaper explosions?

It can be very difficult to empathize with their drama when you have an actual, real life to care for day in and day out. The stories nonparent friends share with you (mind you, this was how you sounded only months prior) sound like noise and ridiculous gossip compared to your "real problems."

I remember trying to maintain eye contact over coffee with friends one day not long after the birth of my daughter. I was the only one who had a child, and I prided myself in the miracle that it was to have gotten up, showered, breastfed the baby, and found matching socks in time to meet them for brunch. My baby was screaming when I left, and although I absolutely knew she was going to be perfectly fine and alive without me for a couple hours, it was all I could do to get her out of my head. I just wanted to enjoy my latte and gab about nonsense like the good ol' days.

I couldn't even focus. At first I could only think and pray about whether Matilda was really okay. I pictured a few irrational scenarios of grand trauma, and after those subsided I determined she must be all right; otherwise, the phone would have rung. By the time I was able to focus on whatever dramatic tale my friends were droning on about, I found myself thinking, "These yahoos are ridiculous! These aren't problems! I've seen worse issues on infomercials, for goodness sake. And I would know! I was up at 4 a.m. watching them when I couldn't get my baby to sleep!"

I don't know whether my friends could see my eyes glazing over that day. But the truth was, I just didn't care about their lives in that moment. It's not fun to admit, but that's how far my perception had skewed into motherhood.

Eventually, as sleep and sanity were slowly restored and I began to let go a little bit more with each time I left my baby in the care of someone else, I was able to focus again on what mattered. Friendships matter. And having a friendship that matters means you care enough to care about what that friend cares about.

Your nonparent friends who care about you might not understand why you fight tooth-and-nail to protect nap time schedules. They might not grasp what it means to forget the pacifier at home or leave a blanket at the mall. And they probably don't care at all whether you got spit-up on your favorite sweater, again. But if they continue listening, if they smile or nod, if they offer to help even if they aren't sure what that means, they're a keeper.

Just do your best to remember to ask them about their world as well. You never know, it may be the closest you'll come to escaping spit-up-land for quite a while.

31

Welcome to the Mom Club

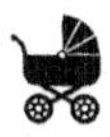

Every new mother experiences multiple births. I don't mean in the infant sense, of course; that is, unless you actually gave birth to more than one baby. If you did, please close this book, pat yourself on the back, and go lie down, sweetheart! You deserve a nap! Rather, I mean that having a baby ushers in all kinds of new features for your new life, none of which can be found on your baby registry.

When you have a baby you also give birth to a new marriage, a new home design, a new schedule—and last but not least—new friendships. Certainly your pre-existing friendships take on new identities of their own, as I addressed in the last chapter. But new people attract new people, and there is just something about a new baby that can't help but attract entirely new people into your fresh world of parenthood.

I'm talking about new mom-friends. Congratulations! You've given birth to an entirely new realm of friendship you never even knew existed until now. You've entered the club. You know the handshake. You have the secret password (it's *coffee*, by the way.) You've all even decided on a nearly-matching wardrobe to set yourselves apart from the rest of society just so everyone can look at you and tell you're from that special sect of women. You are in the Mom Club.

Mom-friends are awesome and annoying and always in competition with each other over something. You can be the most peaceful person on the planet, but when the gloves come off and the labor stories start rolling, you'd better be ready to up the ante and exaggerate the hell out of how many excruciating hours your perfect little angel put you through.

Mom-friends want one thing and one thing only, and they will gripe or weep or giggle until they get it: validation. What's uglier is that no matter how much you try, you can't help but get sucked into the race and get greedy when someone starts handing out tissues or cookies or compliments. You're too tired and insecure to care. You just want a hug and a nap like everyone else. Welcome aboard! You've just experienced your first round of "Show and Tell," Mom-Club style.

Mom-friends are a whole new kind of friend. Unlike any other, they start as soon as you make the grand announcement that you're pregnant. You may as well have a banner hanging over your head saying "Happy Initiation!" as you are welcomed into the club, spending the next nine months paying your dues to most decidedly confirm your membership.

Momdom is the utmost—or should I say the mother of—all sororities. You have amazing, essential support unlike anywhere else, but there is also room for judgment and insecurity. It may take a while for you to get your bearings or feel comfortable, but once you find your clique you'll be just fine.

There are a lot of different kinds of moms out there. I noticed this right away. Each mom I met had her own individual experience of pregnancy, birth, and then motherhood, which expanded into endless stories of parenting anecdotes. These new mom-friends seemed to flock to me out of nowhere. Of course, I hadn't been seeking them out prior to conceiving, so once my bump started to grow and word got around, I suppose we all just sort of found each other.

Here is the great thing: mom-friends get it, for the most part, anyway. Mom friends are empathetic, understanding, and great resources of advice for all things from a plugged milk duct to how to get Desitin out of carpet. They have a story (or ten) for every incident you can come up with, they smile at you even if you haven't showered, and they don't care if you've hung up on them in the middle of a conversation because your baby just woke up or threw up on you. They are relatively forgiving, they are extraordinarily sympathetic, and they can offer a lot of support just by sharing the sheer common bond of motherhood. Mom-friends are essential to quality parenting. Get them. You need them.

Mom-friendships are like college, though—you get out of them what you put into them. They are unlike any other friendships I've had in the past, because we're all sharing this dynamically unique exchange of unpredictable circumstances. Each experience is the same and yet vastly different. We're all climbing the same mountain but taking totally different routes to get there. Some of us might be in better shape than others. Some of us might encounter terrible weather. But all of us want the same thing when we reach the top: happy, successful, productive children who grow up to make a difference, know God, and thank us in the end. Okay, that last part might be a bit idealistic, but hey, a mother can dream too.

ALL ROADS LEAD THERE

Mom-friendships start even before the baby comes because, as you may already know, that journey takes different routes as well.

We first started trying to conceive at the same time two of my other friends and their husbands did. It's an odd and intimate thing to share with a friend that you're "trying" and all, so it was nice to have a sort of secret bond with these two gals as we all took the leap toward the same goal at the same time. It was like cliff diving together—not sure what awaited us below and all a little scared of what we might find.

Not three weeks in, I got a call from one of the friends. Sure enough, on their first try, their first night, their first cycle, they got pregnant. Wow! I was shocked and elated for her. It had just barely sunk in for me that I was ready for this next giant step in life, so while I had a smidgen of jealousy, I hadn't even had a chance to think about it long enough to worry. I was just enjoying the idea of it all, so it didn't strike me as anything but good news when she called to tell me.

Then the months dragged on. The other friend and I were still waiting on our good news. I watched my pregnant friend grow and grow, finally give birth, and even send out her birth announcements before I even got pregnant. But then it was my turn, and suddenly I was the one making the call to the nonpregnant friend with my news. I just couldn't do it. What would I say? How would she react?

I decided if I was going to do it, I was going to do it right. I didn't want to feel bad or guilty about being happy, but I didn't want to make her feel any worse than she already did. I bought her a dozen roses, asked her to come over, and told her in person honestly, quickly, and followed by a hug. It was awkward. It was weird. It was uncomfortable . . . and totally the best thing ever.

I had a really difficult and honest communication process with this friend over those following nine months. I wanted to be sensitive to her fertility issues and yet be completely ecstatic for myself at the same time. I wanted to gush about my belly and new baby clothes and colors for the nursery. But more importantly, I wanted to be the kind of person who could be told to shut up and can it before I made my friend feel about as big as a ladybug. I wanted to keep my friend, so I kept the dialogue between us going, awkward or not.

About a year and a half after all that, my friend adopted the most beautiful baby girl. Now we're great mom-friends, just as we were great nonmom-friends before. But it wasn't easy. I'm sure there were days she wanted to punch me in the face for complaining about morning sickness. There were days my feelings were hurt because she didn't ask me how I was doing. I'm sure there were times we avoided each other a little bit because our routes up the mountain didn't feel fair one way or the other, but we were making it work and high-fiving each other along the way as best we could.

Supportive mom-friends are key to sustaining your sanity.

I find it essential to all other avenues in my life to have a supportive group of women who can relate to what I'm going through and can listen to my life's burdens and joys without judgment. But, as I said before, it's all give and take. You have to invest in these kinds of relationships in order to receive the kind of support you are longing for and definitely needing.

I say definitely because, let me tell you, I know a LOT of moms, and not one of them has ever bragged to me about how they're doing this whole parenting thing spectacularly on their own and without the support of anyone else. It's not possible. It doesn't just take a village to raise a child anymore; it takes a family, a church, an online community, a Twitter following, a few mom blog forums, at least four friends you text daily, a weekly phone call to your mother, a monthly date night with your husband, and three or four fairly-worn parenting books on your night stand (not to mention a quality travel mug and a reliable vacuum.) And we're still all complaining about never getting enough rest!

32

Social Media and the Modern Mama

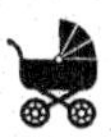

Local mom-friends are not your only resource for friend support. I'm gonna take a stab in the dark (call me crazy here) but I'm guessing you probably have a Facebook account. Most of us do, and I'm no exception. I frequently peruse the news feed scouring for updates related to parenting. If I've had a rough day, it can feel great to spot someone else's status update about how they also got three hours of sleep or their kid woke up with the flu. On the contrary, when a fellow mom-friend is out on the town and Instagrams a sweet pic of herself in her date-night best, I feel happy to know my friends are escaping the wiles of needy babes for the night. Facebook and other online media can be a brief, sweet, mental escape as well as a resource for boosting motivation or just connecting with fellow moms (and obviously other friends too.)

But, warning to the wise, don't be deceived by the constant flow of good-looking photos and updates that might make your life feel drab and boring. Facebook can be a breeding ground for insecurities as well, so be careful.

THE ILLUSION OF A PERFECT LIFE

When I've had a long day, get home from work and find my baby screaming at the top of her lungs, the last thing I want to see on Facebook is how some mom might be doing it all better than me. Know what I'm saying here? At the end of the night, when I'm exhausted and totally at a loss as to how I will wake up and do it all again the next day, it can feel very defeating to go online and view the perfectly-filtered Instagram photos of my fellow mom-friends looking fantastic.

It's a modern-day fairy tale; that's all it is. It's an illusion. It's pretty and inviting but not a reflection of actual life. Chances are real good that photo of your friends's new baby wearing the hair bow and sitting next to her toy poodle all went haywire two seconds after the flash went off. You rarely see the blurry photos of a screaming newborn who just pooped all over her Christmas dress, but you know it happens. That's all I'm saying.

Mom-friends want to share the best of the best with you and sometimes the worst of the worst if they can get a rise in sympathy. But the rest of their normal life is almost exactly like yours—laundry, dishes, diapers, vacuum, repeat. Just because someone uses a warm-and-fuzzy filter on their Facebook page doesn't mean they're a better parent than you. You're not alone in sometimes feeling like you don't know what you're doing and everyone else does! It's not true. We're all only saved by the grace of God each and every day. That's the only filter we really need to make our lives all nice and cozy.

I decided a long time before pregnancy to try and live my life as transparently as possible. Pursuing the transparent life doesn't mean you're brutally honest all the time or going around exposing inappropriate information or even expressing emotions as you have them without consideration of your surroundings. No, that's not what I'm trying to achieve.

Rather, I think pursuing a transparent life is simpler than that. It's the outward approach to telling the world I don't accept myself, but Jesus does. Then it becomes just about seeking Jesus, accepting my belonging to Him and His care for me, and living my life accordingly. In other words, my actions and words flow from my motivation to become more like Jesus.

When I said I don't accept myself, I could almost audibly hear some of you gasp in sympathy. Didn't you? You wanted to jump in and hug me or make sure I'm okay or feeling good. But then you'd be missing the point.

My accepting myself does me no good. My accepting my belonging to Jesus saves me completely. Think about this. What can I do for me? Compliment myself with kind thoughts? You can do that for me, too. Remind myself about my skills or accomplishments? The fruit of my labor does that for me.

Think back to the selfishness spectrum, how I am at my best the more devoid of myself I become and the more filled with the love of Christ I am. My belonging to Jesus and allowing His acceptance of me, His forgiveness for me, His grace upon me, is only visible the more transparent I become (and here you thought I was using the term figuratively the whole time!) Through my weaknesses, which I willingly bring to light, Christ's strength is made evident. This is pursuing the transparent life, for me.

This belief became fundamental to my understanding of parenthood, because right out of the starting gate it felt like I didn't know what I'd gotten myself into. I believed I would be a good mother. There was no other option. I *would* be a good mother, so help me!

DON'T GO IT ALONE

I had been blessed throughout my life to encounter many, many good mothers along the way. I would pick up tidbits of wisdom here and there, filing them away for future use. I would also silently judge parents, just as every single nonparent out there does, making blanket statements in my head like *I would never say that to a child* or *I won't do that when I have a baby* and so forth.

But it's all entirely different and frightening when you're holding your own baby—the one person who is going to actually be influenced by this accumulation of advice, and you suddenly feel at a loss for what to do. Here's what you do: you ask for help.

Asking for help is an absolute *must* in the pursuit of a transparent life. In fact, if you are a follower of Christ, it is essential to faith alone that you recognize your complete need for Jesus, therefore admitting you cannot help yourself. Why is it, then, that the next logical step—asking for help—feels so entirely gruesome and unbecoming?

Pride.

It sounds silly when you're talking about diaper duty or midnight feedings, but trust me when I tell you there is more to it than it seems. At some point in parenthood—and this is most likely going to hit you a lot sooner than you imagine—you are going to hit a wall and not know what to do. Maybe it will be about diapers. Maybe it will be about midnight feedings. And maybe it will be about something more, like how you can't talk to your husband about anything other than the baby or you don't feel like you connect to your newborn or you just feel ugly since coming home from the hospital.

It's never too late to lay down your pride, humble yourself, and ask for help. Start with a prayer, ask God for confidence and faith in Him, then seek out a trusted source for honest feedback or dependable advice. And remember, you aren't supposed to already know what you don't know.

33

Change the Baby, Not the Husband

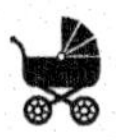

When my husband and I brought our baby girl home for the first time, he had never changed a diaper in his life. He was nervous and pretty freaked out to suddenly take part in something he knew had just literally become part of his daily routine overnight. He wasn't without preparation. We had taken the Baby Care 101 class offered through the hospital, and I had shown him a few tricks I learned from being an aunt for years. I knew he could get the hang of it, but it was still he who had to just go for it. And what do you know? Within weeks he was a total diaper-changing champ.

That didn't come as any surprise to me. I knew—before ever seeing him change her diaper—that my husband would be able to care for our daughter, poo-splosions and all. We had talked about it and he was very open about asking for help, whatever the task may be, and telling me when he didn't know something or understand something about basic baby care. He was engaged, involved, and even read some chapters of the half dozen parenting books I stacked up on our bookshelf over the course of the pregnancy.

What did come as a surprise to me was my lack of humility. I guess I was so busy making sure I was prepared for what was coming (overly prepared, perhaps) that I never saw it coming. Pride, that is. Baby care aside for a moment, I had never been a wife to a new daddy who didn't know anything about babies. I had never before taught someone (again and again and again) how to hold or change or bathe or swaddle a newborn before. So, as much help as I was in the caring-for-a-newborn department, I all but failed when it came to the being-patient-with-a-learning-new-father department.

I needed help. Not in the usual way this time. Not in the way most new mothers do when they end up calling their nurse at midnight asking why the baby won't latch on or what to do when diaper rash won't go away. No, I needed advice on how to extend inordinate amounts of grace to my eager-to-help husband who was often causing more mischief than good! I struggled with allowing him the freedom to learn in his own time, in his own way.

Before the baby came, I would have thought there was no way on Earth I would feel that way. I thought I would be so grateful to just have him around that I couldn't imagine getting frustrated with him. But when you're running late to meet friends and you're blow-drying your hair and your husband is taking twenty minutes to change the baby when you know you could have done it in about three . . . you are real close to blowing a gasket and running your mouth off at that oh-so-endearing heart of his, wanting to help out and all. Let's face it—it's in our nature as women to jump ahead and do things for ourselves. Surely, it was a woman somewhere talking about her husband who came up with the famous phrase *If you want it done right, you have to do it yourself!*

Dear me, I did not want to turn into that woman! (More on how to avoid that potential disaster in the next chapter.)

But I'm sorry to tell you that my pride got the better of me. Pride, lack of sleep, and poor time management, anyway. I didn't seek out advice. I didn't ask any of my close friends about how I should deal with stuffing a boatload of impatience down my throat (don't do that, by the way.) I didn't open up and just lay it out there for someone to come along and say "How 'bout you give this guy a break!"

I should have. And I'm lucky that I was probably too tired to do too much harm to the poor fellow. But by the time I got around to being awake long enough to notice how hard I was being on him, I really started to pray about it. I am so thankful to a Holy Spirit with Whom I can be honest and complain to and vent to about any and every thing and Who never gets tired of hearing from me. With God's grace, I was gradually motivated to start shutting my mouth and become my husband's cheerleader instead of his coach.

It wasn't until months afterward, when I really started to get the hang of allowing my husband the freedom to be the parent he was capable of being, that I heard a friend talk about this same issue. I was thinking in the back of my head "Me too!" and that is the first time it struck me (duh) I should have said something so long ago. I should have asked for advice. I should have opened up, as simple or silly as it may have appeared, and allowed myself to be slapped in the face with some good old-fashioned wisdom.

YOU AREN'T EXPECTED TO KNOW EVERYTHING

Parenting is a constant balance of weeding through solicited and unsolicited advice. But it all starts with the initial admission of not knowing everything, which can be harder than it sounds. After all, if we admit how much we don't know as parents, doesn't it beg the question of just how much our own parents didn't know when they raised us? Funny and scary, isn't it?

The entire first year of parenthood is a grand shock to the system about how much our parents (and all parents we encounter, I would bargain) fly by the seat of their pants when it comes to making decisions. For several months after having Matilda, I felt I was a swinging pendulum, on one side asking loads of questions and getting as much information as possible and then swinging entirely the other direction and abandoning all knowledge for the sake of just getting done whatever task needed to be accomplished.

Who cares if I'm not supposed to give her the pacifier except for nap-time? She's screaming—give her the pacifier! Who says I can't keep her in the crib an extra twenty minutes while I get the laundry folded? What do you mean, I can't give the baby green beans yet? She loves them—let her eat!

Sometimes you just have to throw caution to the wind and figure it out for yourself. Other times you have to keep asking for help until you find a truly sympathetic ear or a genuine response that lends you the best solution.

There is one guarantee, however. With parenthood comes *plenty* of advice.

34

Unsolicited Advice and the Art of Ruining Your Kid

Unsolicited advice is probably the secondary reason (just after pride, that is) why it can seem so gosh-darn difficult to ask for help. You can feel crippled by information overload so easily that to turn around and ask a question can feel like you are back in school, asleep at your desk, only to wake up and ask a question the teacher already answered. *Whoops, I mean, I totally already knew that—just kidding!* Right?

Advice comes from every direction. Friends want to make sure you don't have it as hard as they did, aunts and sisters want to relive their experiences through you, and moms want to make sure you don't screw up your kid like they screwed you up (all the while seeking out validation for the way they parented you.) Everyone just wants to make sure you have everything you need and can do this the best way possible—their way.

It is wonderful to have supportive friends and family. Wonderful. But support is much different than pressure, and that's really important to understand. Support lifts up, holds, makes stronger. Pressure weakens, burdens, and often leads to volatile explosions.

YOU CAN'T PLEASE EVERYONE

You can't please everyone. You won't please someone. You aren't going to do something the "right" way no matter how you do it. Parenting is just too variable an art for someone not to be offended at how you choose to guide your child.

Some moments are going to require a soft *thank you* and smile, followed by quick disregard of their suggestion. Other times are going to necessitate a need for boundaries to be made, actions to be taken, or conversations to be had regarding how "This is my family" and "This is why we do things this way," followed by prayer and an understanding that you can't allow for criticism in particular areas of your life from particular people in your life.

Sometimes advice from others (especially unsolicited advice) can turn very serious or dramatic very quickly, so I would encourage you to proceed with compassion when responding to others' suggestions (flippant or not.) Oftentimes, when people offer an opinion you didn't ask for, it's because they deeply value it or were hurt in the past due to the nature of whatever topic they are addressing. Keep this in mind when you feel the urge to brush off what people tell you. Sometimes the simple phrase *I'll keep that in mind* can be enough to appease their helpful spirit and allow you to move on from the conversation.

Try not to assume people are judging your parenting skills as much as you think they are. They probably aren't. And if they are, they probably won't tell you. And if they do, then please revert back to "I'll keep that in mind" and pray for them. Chances are good their judgments have far more to do with their own insecurities or history than they have to do with your shortcomings.

It won't take long before you'll catch yourself becoming the one to hand out the advice, solicited or not. Maybe even when you're still pregnant (if you are so bold) you will begin to extend the helpful hand of opinion giving (what a gift!) and let it be known why you are making the choices you are making. (Ha! If you are reading this book, you understand the facetious tone and irony of my last sentence!)

It's true. I've always had plenty to say and have rarely feared handing out my own take on what I think about this or that. Pregnancy and parenthood have not been spared my observations. But I had a lot of advice and information coming to me throughout my pregnancy, and it was hard to stomach some of the more condescending suggestions that came my way.

TAKE IT OR LEAVE IT

I can't tell you how many times we had friends who were already parents themselves tell us "Sleep now, because you'll need it!" or "Go see a movie now, because you won't after the baby comes!" or "Enjoy your time as a couple, because it will never be the same!" And every time we would nod, roll our eyes, and try our best to laugh it off. It seemed so silly to us, like we could even store up sleep or movies or time if we wanted to.

After the baby was born, the condescension continued. "Enjoy that sleeping newborn now before she starts to crawl!" or "Just wait until she learns to talk!" or "Be thankful for that special time when you first bring her home!"

It got to the point where I just wanted to tell those people to go jump in a lake already. *Like I'm not thankful enough? I can't ever just enjoy my baby already? Get off my back!*

It wasn't long after we brought our new baby home that some of our other friends were announcing their own pregnancies. Just like engagements in college or wedding announcements when you first join the workforce, we had officially entered that phase of life when, one after another, our couple friends were turning up pregnant. Babies, babies, babies.

And guess what we started to tell all of them? "Sleep! Sleep now! You'll never sleep again!" "Travel while you can! Enjoy your couplehood!" As soon as those babies were born, guess what we couldn't shut up about? "Oh, your baby is so precious. Eat up this sacred time because it slips away so quickly. Just don't take it for granted." And "Enjoy the calm, quiet newborn phase before they turn into raving, moving lunatics who cause mess wherever they go. Oh, and here's a casserole. Good luck!"

Yup. It happened. The condescendees had become the condescenders. *Wah waah.*

It wasn't for quite some time after dishing out this spiel to our friends that I realized what had happened. I think I audibly cringed when it hit me. But then, in all honesty, I had to just shrug and laugh about it. They were right! We were right! It was all so true.

35

The Paradox of Parenthood

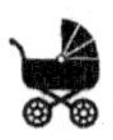

Babies are like time machines. Life goes at a normal, decent pace for decades, and then all of a sudden you bring a new life into the world and warp speed throttles you forward into an unfamiliar era you never anticipated. You want it all to soar by and slow down all at the same time. You want to know you'll survive it, but you also want to soak it up and make the most of it. You want to see that it all turns out okay, that you did a good job and everyone made it out alive and well, and in the same breath you never want anything to change. Parenthood isn't just emotional; it's physiological, sentimental, and spiritual.

You just helped create a person you will know eternally. How often does that happen in a lifetime? How many people can you say you were there for when they entered this world? How many can you truly promise to be there for until one of you departs from this world?

Once you experience something as transcending as parenthood, you can't help but want to shout from the rooftops about how it has affected your life. I've felt this way about Jesus. I've felt this way about marriage. And now, I've felt this way about a tiny little baby who will forever be part of my life.

How can I not want to hold on to that sort of energy and pass on all I know about it if I think it can help someone else understand it a little more clearly?

This is exactly why all those crazy parents before me wanted to get my attention and make sure I knew what I was getting myself into. It's exactly what motivated them to stop me in my tracks and get me to appreciate the depth of what I was about to encounter, not only what was ahead of me, but what was going to be behind me too. They wanted me to make sure I knew that the life I was leaving behind was forever lost (though absolutely worth the exchange) and what was ahead was to be revered, respected, and remembered.

Here's the catch: There's no way for someone to learn this without experiencing it. Just like Jesus, just like marriage, having a baby is an experience untouchable by words or ideas. It can't be explained completely, anticipated wholly, or understood entirely until it is within your grasp.

If this sounds dramatic, good. It is! It's about as grand and dramatic as life gets!

Still, knowing that it takes someone experiencing the entire process for them to appreciate condescending suggestions like "Sleep more" or "Be grateful" doesn't necessarily keep them from coming out of my mouth. Like myself, I think all new parents live in the fog of infatuation with each new phase of life we are experiencing.

When I was pregnant, I was afraid I wouldn't love having the baby as much as I loved having her inside me. When she was first born, I was worried I would miss her snuggly little body if she grew any bigger. When she started to move a bit, I worried I wouldn't love her as much when she started walking. Now, I worry she'll be harder to love the farther down the road we go.

Yet each new phase has brought two things with it: brief grieving for the loss of what was and incredible joy for what is. The love I have for her only grows. It shouldn't be surprising to me, but it always is. The boundaries of what I believe I'm capable of—how I'm capable of loving her—expand beyond each new phase life brings.

WHERE IS THAT PAUSE BUTTON, ANYWAY?

Do I miss the newborn stage? Parts of it, sure. Would I trade any part of the present for a moment of the past? Not a bit. After all, the present will be the past of the future, and I wouldn't want to miss it for a second. Although we might have 20/20 hindsight and wish we could utilize a time machine to tell your nonpregnant self to fully engage in each moment with the fullest extent of gratitude, it just isn't possible. We can't go back in time. We can't re-thank our past pleasures. We can't relive our former freedoms. And we certainly can't cash in on any sleep we may have previously stored up no matter how many naps we may have taken in our youth. But we can live and breathe and speak our gratitude for the present and do the best we can to encourage those around us to do the same.

You may roll your eyes at some of my advice now, but I'll venture a guess you'll be joining the crowd of condescenders sooner than you might think! And welcome aboard. Let's shake hands, call a truce, and just hug it out for a minute. There are still an awful lot of future surprises left in our lives to unknowingly take plenty for granted right now! (Cheers to that!)

36

Playing the Baby Card

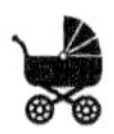

This brings me to my need for spiritual support, specifically as it pertains to parenthood. It's imperative to my well-being. Not just my mental health, my emotional state, but simply as a system of accountability set into motion that keeps me actively seeking Jesus in a real and honest way. This sounds formal, but relax, I'm not going to ask you to get out your highlighters and do an inductive Bible study with me (those are great, by the way, but I've always found them a bit stuffy and intimidating.)

I'm talking about relationships, church, fellowship, Bible reading, counseling, mentorship, and stewardship. How are you going to balance all of this when you can hardly remember what your name is after a night of teething and nursing? You are. You will. You must.

Of all the things in your life that are tempting to let slip, this is going to be one of the easiest. Right after you deliver, you're going to worry about your baby, then your husband, then yourself, and that is followed by a flurry of thoughts ranging from "What's for dinner?" to "How will I get my waistline back?" and everything in between.

Somewhere amidst all that are your questions about God, Jesus, Christian parenting, and how everything you ever thought you knew might be on the brink of deconstruction once you start to realize you are slowly imposing it upon your sparkling-new and perfect baby human who is as innocent as a newly-fallen snowflake. Yikes!

Don't deny these thoughts or distract yourself from them! They are real; they are honest; they are healthy! But let me warn you now, you won't know the answers to most of these daunting inquiries. And that's okay. You're not supposed to. What is important is that you allow yourself the freedom to think about them, to ask God about them, and to engage with others about them as well. This is what it feels like to actively participate in growing up—both the growing up of yourself *and* your now-developing-by-the-minute child.

It seems so easy to disengage from deeper questions about God and your relationship with Jesus when you have a needy baby screaming right in front of you. On the other hand, it can feel like you are in the presence of something genuinely heaven-sent when you hold your child and stare at the miracle she is. Even that can be a distraction from what your soul is yearning for. Just sitting next to miracles is not what Jesus has called us to do.

HOW TO GET OUT OF JUST ABOUT ANYTHING AND WHY YOU SHOULDN'T

Having a baby is a perfect excuse to get out of just about anything. You can run late for work, get-togethers, even bow out of formal invitations when you have a new baby to blame. No one is going to question your priorities when you put the wee one first. No one is going to judge you (at least, not to your face) when you place the needs of your child above other values. And, by all means, when your child is in genuine need, certainly she should help dictate the order of events in your life. Just be careful not to abuse playing the "baby card."

Going to church can easily slip into the "chore" category when you are desperate for a day off. Skipping Bible study can feel mandatory after having your mind taxed between work and marriage and parenthood. Fellowship with Christian friends (even those including words like "potluck" or "cookie exchange") can seem more like a trap brewing up nothing more than guilt or obligation inside of you.

And so now that you have that baby and all . . . you just don't go.

Let me tell you, excuses come easy but they won't be worth it. It's like I told a friend of mine one day, "If you think life is easy, you're doing it wrong." I'm all for the occasional convenience. I think we can agree there have been times we've praised Jesus for sending us McDonald's or duct tape or even Tide pens. Sometimes there is just nothing better than to take a shortcut and get a quick fix as we move along on our merry way. But, if I *only* ate McDonald's, I'd probably be fat. If I *only* used duct tape, half my living room would fall apart. If I *only* used Tide pens, my clothes would smell terrible. Shortcuts just won't cut it all the time. You can't live on shortcuts, nor would you want to.

So why would we think our spiritual life would be any different?

YOUR FIRST STEP, NOT YOUR LAST RESORT

It's funny (sort of) but I don't know how many times I've had a problem arise (really, it could be any kind of issue) and I've found myself frustrated because I couldn't fix it and couldn't figure out why, only to finally take it to the Lord in prayer and have the clouds part over my heart about the matter. Time and again I'm reminded how I need to make prayer my first step and not my last resort. This doesn't mean prayer solves all my problems; of course it doesn't work that way. But taking it to the Throne and relinquishing control over a matter lightens my heart. And remembering not to bear the burden takes practice. In other words, only stopping to ask God for what I really need or trying to maintain communication just when I'm so bogged down I can't handle it on my own . . . well, that's just not enough! Yes, I am enough just as I am for Jesus. He will never turn His back on me, and He is faithful even when I am unfaithful (Hallelujah!) But I'm not an acquaintance to Jesus. I'm His child. I'm in deep. I'm completely His. My entire identity is found within Him. How am I supposed to get by in life if I'm only checking in with Him when I think I need Him?

That's just human foolishness. The fact is I always need Him. This is a beautiful, wonderful thing! It's only a surprise to me when I'm in the thick of a new issue and pondering and worrying myself to death over a matter when, as if a light bulb lights up over my brain, it dawns on me to hand it over to Jesus. This is why it becomes so important to counter our daily routine (our comfortable, natural selves) with spiritual impositions.

It may seem easy to disregard church or other fellowship opportunities after you have a new baby because it simply interrupts your already-difficult-enough-to-adjust-to new life. Indeed! Yes! That is the point!

Church, Bible studies, fellowships, and any other Jesus-centered, Spirit-driven, life-improving get-together is absolutely supposed to interrupt our natural, comfortable life. Otherwise, we'd be tempted to just lazily continue on our way, slipping closer and closer into self-indulgent, totally convenient, pleasure-seeking zones of comfort. It's only natural to want to drift towards what feels good and easy.

I'm not advocating you jam your schedule and over commit yourself. Like every other part of life, there's a healthy balance you need to maintain. I'm urging you to guard yourself against the comfort of staying home and backing out of opportunities for spiritual growth and maintenance simply because people are offering you a "pass" with your newly-found parenthood.

FINDING SUPPORT FROM MORE THAN YOUR SPANX

Pace yourself, set boundaries where you must, but don't completely disengage from your Christian community. On the contrary, if there were ever a time to feast on the bounty the Father has placed around you, now is the time, my friend! You are depleted. You are overworked. You are tired. You are starving. Now is the time to get yourself to the table and ask for seconds and even thirds. Fill up that belly like a bear out of hibernation. Nourish your soul and seek Jesus like a new believer! You're going to need all the spiritual energy you can muster when it comes to passing on what you've learned. Never be satisfied with enough. Never put your fork down. It's like taking part in a feast of knowledge that has no end. I like to think of Jesus smiling like the loving parent at the head of the table, authoritative, kind, and joyously offering as much as we can take in serving by serving, encouraging us to pass down however much we can spare to the next person. And there is always more. There is always enough. And we are always, always welcome.

That's one diet you can scratch off your post-pregnancy to-do list! Who would want to starve when you can delight in such a banquet? Taking steps toward your own spiritual growth as a parent is just as essential as learning to breastfeed your infant or bathe your baby properly. It's just that the hospital doesn't offer any free classes on it.

DON'T FORGET ABOUT DADDY

Not only will engaging in your faith help you preserve a healthy mind, body, and spirit; it will nurture your marriage as well. Marriage? Oh yeah, remember that guy? The one you call "husband?" Or at least, you used to call him husband before you started calling him "Daddy." Turns out he's more than just the guy who takes turns changing the baby or warming up the bottles, though sometimes it can be real easy to forget. Turns out all those worries and issues a new mom deals with . . . well, a whole bunch of those have to do with that guy. That wonderful guy. That wonderful, wonderful . . . what's his name again?

Right.

Marriage is the ultimate friendship. So ultimate, in fact, it deserves a whole chapter all its own.

37

The Magical Transformation From Husband to Hero

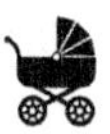

Remember Team Pardy? That idealistic couple who held each other's hand through thick and thin, through boredom and excitement, through uncertainties and new beginnings? Well, by the time we'd been through the ringer of conceiving a baby, off to the races of having a baby, and en-route to raising that baby . . . well, we barely had the energy to spell *Team Pardy*, let alone cheer for it. Whew! Team who again, and what the . . . how's that now?

Bearing a child temporarily took its toll on our marriage, that's for sure. But our value system remained intact through and through. And because of an amazingly supportive community, a diligent (albeit annoying at times) devotion to honest communication, and a gracious God who kept us crazy about each other the whole time, we came out on the other side of pregnancy a stronger and better team than we had ever been before (not to mention we had an additional player in our bracket now!)

Still, the season of baby brought new challenges and obstacles, and neither of us quite knew what to expect. The bad news and the good news here is that both of us were quite honest and up front about not having any idea how to handle it. That being said, we played for the same team, so we were all in either way! I figured if we were able to maintain that perspective, we really couldn't lose.

Team Pardy, play on!

MEETING MICKEY MOUSE

Leaving home as a couple and coming home as a family is one of the more surreal moments of my life. It kind of reminds me of going to Disneyland for the first time. It's nothing like you expected but there is something familiar to it, yet it's more wonderful than you ever imagined.

The first time I went to Disneyland, I was a freshman in college. Since I was going to school in Southern California, many of my friends had already been to Disneyland numerous times, several of them having grown up with it right in their own backyard. But for me, a farm girl from Kansas, it wasn't just an amusement park to kill an hour as a break from homework. To me, it was a magical land where dreams came true.

Growing up, my parents had always wanted to take me and my siblings to Disneyland. They were very generous parents, always planning family trips and summer vacations to make sure we got away from home, had fun, and got to experience some of what American culture had to offer. We took lots of great trips and little outings, and I have fabulous memories of seeing Mount Rushmore and going to water parks in the summer or even camping out with our church at a nearby lake every fall. But I never met Mickey Mouse.

I can remember years when the Disneyland brochures would be scattered across our dining room table. I would stare at the photos and dream about sunny, colorful days filled with cotton candy and giant cartoon characters. We would all get our hopes up, praying that the harvest was good, praying that this would be the year I could see the Magic Kingdom for myself and return to school wearing my Mickey Mouse ears and gush to my friends about our amazing adventure. But time and money came and went, and before we knew it, everyone had grown up and moved on.

Don't feel sorry for me. I recognize it is an insane privilege to even be able to travel at all with family. I see now how spoiled I was to vacation whatsoever. Seriously, I get it now as an adult. But I will be honest that my seven-year-old self had zero perspective (duh) and only thought about her dreams being passed over year after year.

So when I finally saw the Magic Kingdom for myself I just couldn't believe it. I mean, it was so . . . so . . . small? But so beautiful! It wasn't exactly what I had expected, but it was also everything I had hoped for. I guess the dream of seeing it had been so deeply implanted in my heart that there was just no way I could be disappointed. Sadness at Disneyland was an impossibility to me, and I loved everything about it immediately, even if it was different than what I had anticipated. Still, to this day, after having been to Disneyland now dozens of times as an adult, I can't watch the fireworks without shedding a tear. The sheer joy of it all overwhelms me, and I'm just a grateful seven-year-old again, standing in awe of a dream coming true.

This is what it felt like to come home from the hospital with our new baby. It was different than what I anticipated, but not disappointing. I didn't necessarily feel like it was a parade of bliss, but the thought of it feeling like anything less than perfect was an impossibility, just as Disneyland had been. Gratitude was my only option, and it ran so deeply through my veins within the moment that I didn't have room to experience any other interpretation of my emotions.

NOT JUST THE TWO OF YOU ANYMORE

We had just had a baby together, he and I. We made her. She was ours.

These thoughts ran like a broken record through my brain. I was so tired, so in love, so happy and confused all at once that I didn't quite know how to translate my new feelings toward my husband. And, let's be honest, if *I* didn't know, then I was certain *he* most likely didn't have a clue how he felt toward me. We had just been through a marathon together. We were in love and full of pride for each other. It had been the accomplishment of a lifetime, and we were bringing home the ultimate prize. Yet all our focus was constrained to this new prize, this tiny little human, and she held our hearts in her hands.

Weren't these hearts *just* ours? Had we not but moments ago held each other's hearts as if to clutch them for all eternity? And then, in one solemn swoop, she had leapt into the world and snatched them from our senses. Just like that, our attention was forever divided. Never again would we be able to look deeply into one another's eyes without the thought of her in our minds. This was a good thing. This was a difficult thing.

Prior to the birth, I had never thought about relinquishing my husband as my priority. I went into parenthood thinking, "Sure, I will love my child, but my husband will always come first. I understand that in order for our family to function correctly, a healthy marriage needs to be the foundation. He must come first." This is true. This is good. This is the kind of thing you hear on Christian radio stations that makes you smile and nod your head and then nag your husband to change in the next sentence. Right?

This promise was really easy to keep before having a baby. He *was* my world and fairly easy to please. We loved each other and wanted to spend time together, so it was only natural to want to continue this focus after the baby was here. But I hadn't met my baby yet when I made that promise. After she was here, I mean, after she was in my arms and I was staring into her big, dark eyes of hope and after I started nursing her and loving her with God-like love . . . well, it was pretty easy to ditch that bozo in the corner who was snoring loudly and totally forsake all my previous intentions.

Yikes. That's harsh. But I'm pretty sure when maternal instinct kicks in, it knows no bounds. It's like this innate response for protection that makes you want to punch everyone in the face who cocks their head slightly at your new child. Motherhood brings upon you this fierce notion that no one will ever love your baby like you do, and therefore no one can provide for her as well or in the same way. It's irrational, yes, but when you hold your baby for the first time, you can't tell me you didn't feel that punch-you-in-the-face gusto that would give anything for your new infant.

What was to become of us? Team Pardy had grown, but the core remained the same. There was a new player, maybe, but we were the owners. We were the decision-makers. We held the power, not her, and as simple or trite as that sounds, it's imperative to comprehend and accept this in order to succeed at marriage after you have a child.

Repeat after me: *I am still the boss.*

This child does not rule your life; make no mistake about it. As much as we tried to prepare for it ahead of time, having a baby is just one of those things you can't quite entirely prepare yourselves for. We had taken a "babymoon" and tried to enjoy as many freedoms as we could imagine prior to her arrival. We had slept as much as we possibly could, though even that becomes a joke at the end as I was creeping out of bed every ninety minutes (literally, you could set a clock by me) to pee for the sake of my ever-pressurized bladder. We couldn't see one more movie, because we had seen them all. There was nothing more to max out on in our couplehood. We were done with being "us" and ready to be a family.

And yet, after she was born, there was a grieving period. Some people might think this morbid or depressing or altogether wrong. But the truth is (as with any major chapter in your life) having a baby is death to your previous life together. I *don't* mean that it is worse. And I *don't* mean to compare it in any way to an actual death (my heavens, no.) But the life of couplehood as you knew it before having a baby is gone forever—never to be had again—at least not like it used to be.

Welcome to your new neighborhood, or should I say New Couplehood—population 3.

FALLING IN LOVE WITH MR. WHAT'S-HIS-NAME AGAIN

When you first arrive home, you're both in survival mode.

Birthing classes might not tell you this, but you will both be in a dazed state of shock and completely overtired and overwhelmed. You will be smiling and nodding and telling people repeatedly that you feel "fine." Yet in the brief seconds you get to yourself (like, painfully using the bathroom now and then) you will discover you might actually want everyone to leave so you can just take a quick nap in the bathtub.

Here's what he's thinking: *Is she okay? Am I doing a good job? Can I sleep now? How many days till we can have sex again? Do any of these thoughts make me a bad father?* And that's pretty much it.

Men are wonderful and wonderfully simple. This is a good thing! God made men so particularly wired that we crazy womenfolk would be able to completely split our focus between caring for a new life and knowing exactly how to make our men happy. In a word, here is what he needs: encouragement.

GIVE CREDIT WHERE CREDIT IS DUE

I can't say exactly how your man best interprets encouragement. I would urge you to figure out his love language and try your best to remember this in the early days of motherhood. When all else fails, straight-up words of affirmation are a fine place to start.

Remember back when I was going crazy and trying to keep my mouth shut about having to teach my husband how to care for our newborn? Not exactly my shining moment as a new mom. But something I learned about my husband (and, I gather, all husbands) through that process was that he is good. I don't know about you, but I didn't marry an idiot. I'm just going to take a stab in the dark and bet you didn't either. He was able to care for himself and make it in this world without my help somehow between the time he left home and met and married me. He is able to survive without my intervention. Sure, he might need some delicate guidance on things like diaper duty or feeding a baby or rocking her to sleep. But your confidence in him will go a *lot* further than your instruction.

So how can I build up the confidence of my husband as a new father? You probably already know the answer: keep him first. It goes back to that lovely, original intention I had right before delivering our child into the world, right before our couplehood was interrupted and altered forever. He is my first priority.

This is a hard one. It's going to be very difficult for some of you. It's not going to be easy for any of you. Babies are neeeeeeedy little people. Crazy needy. And they are relentless when it comes to screaming and batting eyelashes of shame. They know exactly how to press your buttons and get you to drop everything for them, no doubt about it.

In my opinion, you can't spoil a newborn. It's impossible. Some grandmother somewhere will tell you otherwise, I'm sure. ("You're holding her too much! You shouldn't let her sleep on you!") But the reality is that new babies need a lot, need it often, and will take as much as they can get. The good news is that newborns actually sleep quite a bit for the first few weeks as well. (Thanks, God!) It's sort of an evil trick, because they sleep fairly well and then all of a sudden they might be up every couple hours, but hey, for that first few weeks it's a lovely ride, so enjoy it.

Since you really can't spoil a newborn, you're going to give in. They cry; you answer. It happens. Cherish it, as this time is short-lived and sacred, and do all you can to just be there in the moment taking a million photographs to chronicle this time for which you will mostly be blurry-eyed and heavily caffeinated.

But after the first several weeks drift by, as you are settling into some sort of new norm and establishing a kind of routine, you will begin to see the fog lift. As the haze clears, you will see a shadowy image emerge, a figure both familiar yet unrecognizable. He is handsome yet worn with experience. He is charming but weary. This is your husband. The new father.

You may need to reintroduce yourself. You've both been through the ringer, and it may have been a while since you stopped to stare into each other's eyes (that is, if you can tear them off your new bundle of joy for a moment.) Aha . . . yes! You recognize him now? The one you love. Your soulmate. And best of all, the man God has given to you to live life with.

YOU ARE STILL A COUPLE

It's time for you to reestablish yourselves as a couple. It will seem too early, I'm sure. After all, those first six weeks fly by, and before you know it, you're back in the stirrups getting the green light from your OB/GYN and frightened with the excitement of wedding-night jitters all over again. This is normal! This is good! This is when you need to take a deep breath, call a girlfriend, have a glass of wine, and start genuinely communicating with your spouse again.

Your world has been nothing but breast milk, casseroles, pacifiers, diapers, and late-night infomercials for the last several weeks. Whew! Not exactly a recipe for romance, if you know what I'm saying. I'm not just talking about sex (though that *is* part of reconnecting and a vital step in initiating yourselves into the realm of couplehood again.) But, more so, I'm talking about taking a "baby time-out" and stopping to wholeheartedly engage with your husband.

Before having a baby, Josh and I had always joked that date night wouldn't really mean anything until after children. It seemed like every night was date night! We lived in the luxury of each other's full attention. We indulged in laziness and eating out. We kept our own schedules and fought off obligations like the plague. Basically, we loved being together, so whether we actually went out to dinner or saved a buck and rented a movie at home, we didn't care as long as we were just hanging out. We knew we took if for granted, because it was just so darn easy!

But we also knew that once being alone together meant having to get a babysitter and carve out time exclusively for each other a new value would be assigned to date night. There is, however, a vast difference between thinking about it and actually having to do it. The truth is, setting up a date night is not easy, and it's even harder when you're exhausted and broke!

After the baby was born, as simple or pitiful as it may sound, my husband and I missed each other. We could do without the excess freedom, the sleep, even the quiet. But we could not continue on without each other. It wasn't long into our new role as parents when it became obvious we were due for a date night.

38

Date Night: Is that Spit-up On My LBD?

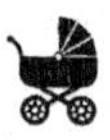

Our anniversary was just three weeks after the baby was born. It seemed wrong not to acknowledge it in some way, but I'll admit I had my reservations about leaving her, if only for a few hours. Luckily, our anniversary always falls close to Thanksgiving, so we had family in town prepared to watch our new baby while we rekindled our sanity . . . er, I mean, romance over a nice dinner.

It was tricky. I completely trusted our family to care for her, to ensure her survival without me, and to accommodate her needs while I was away. But it didn't make any difference when I walked out the door in my cute shoes and Spanx up to my collarbone. I missed her as soon as I closed the door. I worried about her as soon as we left. I felt sorry to have left our family with the burden that so distinctively seemed like my sole responsibility.

We sat down to dinner and gazed into each other's eyes. We sighed deeply, he out of contentment and me out of sheer need for more oxygen. *Was she okay? Did she need me? Is she crying? Does she miss me? Does she think I abandoned her?*

Turns out, these are all completely normal thoughts when you leave your baby for the first time. But knowing you're being irrational doesn't make your feelings any less real. I couldn't focus. I couldn't give my husband my entire attention. I couldn't turn off the motherhood I had just barely, recently, wholeheartedly gotten used to. It helped to change the setting, to get out of the house and into public where other adults gathered and had conversations about more than just feedings and nap schedules. But, again, I took myself wherever I went, and I was a mother in every setting now.

As soon as we returned a mere two hours later, my heart was at ease. She had survived. Better yet, she had slept through the entire thing! Figures. For a few minutes I rolled my eyes at myself and wondered why I had even bothered to go. What was the point of getting all dolled up and getting out there only to worry and pretend the whole time?

Then one look at my husband as we crawled into bed that night, and I knew the answer—him. He loved me. He had seen me, recognized me, and remembered that I wasn't just a new mother; I was his wife. He had been able to check his concerns at the door, leave the baby completely in the care of others, because he so desired to spend time with *me*. Did he care any less about our baby than I did? Of course not. Did he patronize me for checking my phone every five minutes while we were out? No.

THE DIFFERENCE IS IN THE WIRING

Men have this gift from God in the way they're wired. They compartmentalize their emotions into organized little boxes that they get down one at a time and use as needed. He needs to be a dad? He pulls out the box full of authority, care, worry, guidance and provision. He needs to be a husband? He pulls out the box of love, leadership, confidence, service and seduction. They do the best they can to use the resources they are given. They might not always know where to turn when they need more of something, but they're awfully good at focusing when tasked to do something specific.

Women—surprise, surprise—are wired entirely differently. We've pretty much consolidated our boxes into one massive junk drawer, and as long as nobody touches it, we know exactly where everything is. Neither way is right or wrong. Neither way is more efficient or more effective. But lots of emotions can get lost in translation when we're trying to multitask our feelings and they're trying to open and close boxes at the speed of lightning to keep up with us. It can all get very confusing very quickly, and we start misinterpreting his efforts for lack of concern. He gets angry. We cry. And the mess continues.

Have I hit a little close to home? Don't worry; turns out you're normal! Normal doesn't mean you have to settle for misinterpretation and hurt feelings. No, no, no. Everyone wants to feel understood here. This is central to communication in marriage, and it's the only way we can get through the chaotic days of early parenthood without feeling unloved, disrespected, or totally useless.

When we got home from our first date, it would have been really easy for me to cry and try to convince him how he just doesn't understand how much of a big deal it was for me to even leave the house without our baby. I could have resented him for having a better time than I did or threatened to not go out again. I could have read his signs of contentment as total invalidation for how I was feeling, and I could have felt guilty for not having a good time, not being there for my baby, and not caring more about what I wanted for myself.

KEEP YOUR EYE ON THE BIGGER PICTURE

By the grace of God, when we got home and finally settled into bed that night, a new feeling swept over me instead of all those oh-so-common womanly waves of emotion that far too often take the reins. I just looked at my husband, and loved how much he loved me. I felt myself stepping back for a second and seeing the bigger picture—*My husband wants to spend time with me alone*. Um, how could I interpret that truth as anything but wholly honorable and exciting? I'd just won the lottery! That's the best news ever!

Satan wants nothing more than to drive a wedge between married folks. What's more, he loathes, hates, and despises happily-married Christians more than anything. Satan is one sneaky devil (literally) so he's not necessarily going to use evil for evil. He can also use good for evil, and that includes babies and date nights. Who would guess that a sweet, little, innocent baby could cause anything but joy between two people in love? And yet the stress, exhaustion, disruption, and doubt that having a child brings into a marriage is often anything but joyful.

Guard yourself. You're on the same team—you two as a couple and your baby.

Recognizing how much he loved me and knowing that as a man he was able to enjoy his time as a husband apart from being a father gave me the perspective of our team as it was meant to be, just as it has always been—Team Pardy! There was no option for letting anything come between us, not outside issues like money, sex, or in-laws, and now not even our own child. We had to fight for this bond. We had to engage with each other and pursue each other. I had to let go of my natural instinct to allow my baby to come first, and I had to trust God and my husband that they both had my best interest (my best life, even) in mind when they made decisions. And that night of our first date, my husband had made the decision to give me his full attention. Not because I earned it or because he didn't care about the baby or because he wanted anything in return, but because it's how he's wired, and it's what he is called to do as my husband.

Even without his knowing it, that night he put our marriage first. He showed me that his value system for our family was intact, and that Team Pardy would rock on. Yes! This motivated me to want more of the same, to want a marriage worth putting first. To want him.

39

The After Midnight Rule

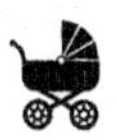

Seeing my husband as my lover again (and not just that guy who took out the diaper trash every day) made me take a closer look at our marriage. But after a few years of marriage and a new baby, things start to get uncomfortably comfortable around the house. That is, it becomes easier and easier to slip into bad habits, put less effort into things, or actually start to resent the familiarity of one's routine.

Idiosyncrasies that were once charming *(He combs his mustache with his fingers when he's trying to think of what to say—so cute!!)* become alarmingly annoying *(He won't stop grooming that stupid mustache with his fingers that he probably didn't even wash after supper—gross!)* And, well, the union between two very different individuals can start to show signs of discord if not attended to immediately.

That being said, marriage can be hard enough at times before children enter the picture. We knew once we encountered this whole, new life-without-regular-sleep situation called parenthood we would need to hold tightly to our vows more than ever. For us, this meant a few new rules had to be established for our sanity (and romance) to sustain the years ahead.

The After Midnight Rule came to be sometime shortly after Matilda arrived. I remember the night well. Matilda was not a good sleeper right from the start. She would cry and fuss and claw at me with relentless and freakish strength I thought only baby grizzly bears could be born with. She wasn't necessarily unhappy . . . she was just *active.* This particular night, the darling child would not shut her eyes. She would not rest.

We were going on only a handful of hours of sleep over the last few days and Josh was trying to push himself through a full-time job during the day, unable to take the occasional catnap that I was attempting to sneak in during daylight. We were exhausted to say the least. The Red Bull and coffee had worn off. The second and third wind had died to a dusty, desert cough.

I remember shushing her and swaying her until my back ached. The soles of my feet were swollen and my eyelids kept springing open and shut like a cartoon window shade. She just kept crying. Finally, I made Josh take over. I was at my limit and I just needed this new daddy to step up to the plate and get this baby to sleep somehow.

I remember lying in bed, too tired to cry. I couldn't help my baby. I didn't know what to do. And Josh wasn't doing any better. He rocked her, he shushed her, he hummed . . . she screamed. The minutes ticked by and suddenly, out of seemingly nowhere, over the top of her cries I heard my husband (my sweet and thoughtful husband, the love of my life and father to my new child) erupt with fierce exclamation "I WANT TO THROW HER THROUGH THE WINDOW!"

I darted out of bed, yanked the screaming babe from his arms and sought haven in the nursery. I burst into tears and rocked the little terror until we were both soaked with our own tears. I couldn't believe it. *Who was that man in the other room and what had he done with my husband?* I was already beyond tired and emotional and had no more wits left to even think about finding their ends. I wanted somebody to rock *me* to sleep and explain who that monster was who was now soundly sleeping in my bed. What had happened to my husband?

I'll tell you what! 2 a.m. and no sleep is what.

By morning, he got ready for work (albeit, groggy looking) but no worse for wear. No explanation, no apology, no remorse. He kissed us both good-bye and left for work, leaving me to wonder if what I had experienced the night before had all been a horrible dream. Is this charming fellow the same jerk who wanted to throw my bundle of joy through the window last night? Am I married to Jekyll and Hyde?

Needless to say, we sorted it out. It took a few talks and a whole lot of coffee, but we came to an understanding that we've found many couples can relate to. Given a highly emotional situation, women tend to resort to emotional responses (crying) and men tend to react with anger. (Yelling, shutting down, or wanting to throw a child through a bedroom window are apparently all natural responses in this situation.)

So what's a couple to do when it's 3 a.m., emotions are running high, and you end up snapping at each other as if you'd never met a worse enemy (and just at the moment when you could really use a partner?) How do you wake up and kiss each other and act like you didn't purposefully throw that pacifier in his face to get him to wake up and get the baby?

Well, we decided right then and there, you do just that. Because nothing after midnight counts. That is the After Midnight Rule. We don't hold anything we say against each other the next morning. Nothing between the hours of midnight to 6 a.m. are begrudged or used to argue a point. It just doesn't count. It can't. We're too tired and we don't mean it. It really is that simple.

Now, when I say simple, don't mistake this for being easy. It's not. There have been many times I can still remember how I felt sad or angry that my husband was not more helpful at two in the morning. I resented the fact that I was blessed with the bosoms to nurse our hungry child in the middle of the night while my beloved snored soundly next to me.

But there also comes to mind many times I was short with him, rude to him, and downright inconsiderate of the fact that he had to get up in a couple hours, present himself as awake and sharp, and go earn a living for which we are both so grateful. So . . . you take a deep breath, you ask God for more grace, you forgive your spouse. Then you go to sleep (eventually) and wake up with a smile and pour them coffee and kiss them good-bye for the day. And you don't bring it up again. Ever.

The After Midnight Rule has even become something of a humorous staple in our home. There have been enough times now that we will actually find ourselves commiserating and even laughing about it in the morning. Sure, maybe we are both just too out-of-our-minds tired to choose arguing over laughing, but that's kind of the point. It just doesn't matter. It really, truly (and believe me, I know this is hard to recall at 3 a.m.) doesn't matter who gets up to get the stupid pacifier for the baby . . . or change her diaper . . . or find that burp rag . . . or change those crib sheets (oh, that's the worst!) Just do it. Or let him. Or whatever the heck will be the most efficient way to get you back to bed as soon as possible—do that. Go to bed angry if you have to. Just go to bed.

And when you wake up in the morning, remember that you hold the potential to set the tone for the day. He's not a monster. He *does* want to help you. He *won't* throw your baby out the window. He needs a hug and some coffee, just like you do.

40

Does This Baby Come With an Instruction Manual?

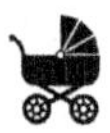

As a new mother, I don't think I anticipated feeling like the expert on my child. But within a few days of being home, it quickly became clear that everyone seemed to default to me on every decision that was made regarding the baby. *Should we feed her now? Has she slept long enough? Do you think she needs a bath?* All questions were directed toward me first, and suddenly I was frightened (and a little flattered) by the amount of power I seized within our home. The baby dictated much of our schedule, and I dictated much of what the baby did; therefore, I had the ability to sway our family with very little effort. It was scary. It was invigorating. It was totally unexpected.

This was a dangerous weapon, this power. Shortly after I realigned my priorities to strive for what God designed, I had a new-found respect for my husband as leader of our family and our home. Just because I loved him, trusted him, and submitted to his ability to lead our family didn't instantly make him any more capable of answering questions like *Is this breast milk too hot in this bottle? Is her car seat fastened tight enough? Should we change her before or after her nap?*

So instead of giving in to a power struggle or endlessly

nagging my husband to be something he's not, I decided to really go out on a limb here and do something extraordinary—trust him.

I know, I know, it sounds crazy. After all, what if he puts her diaper on backwards or feeds her until she throws up or uses too much soap in her hair at bath time? Wait, seriously? What if he *what*?

The best thing I could do for my husband as a new father was to allow him the freedom to be the best dad he was striving to be. I needed to encourage him, to be his helpmate as I was directed and designed to be, and to love him for it (not in spite of it.)

If you want to see a competent, supportive, confident new father, then you as the wife need to encourage the help you want by being the helpmate he needs. He is going to mess up. He's going to put too much diaper cream on or pair up a skirt with a sweatshirt and boots in the middle of summer. He might let her watch too much TV or eat too much applesauce. Maybe he doesn't read to her with the same voices you do or sing the songs you do. But you know what? He's building his own stories, his own memories, his own special bonds with his new baby. And unless you fear it may endanger one or both of them, you have no reason to intervene. Besides, we are called his *help*mate, not his my-way-or-the-highway-mate.

As I said before, I didn't marry an idiot. I didn't marry someone unable to ask for help if he needed my assistance (hey, some diapers just call for backup; let's be honest!) I didn't marry someone who would choose the easier route over the right one. The more I believed this, the more I trusted him. The more I trusted him, the more I believed it.

Men have a tendency to step up to the plate and show us all they're made of when we step back and give them the chance. Sure, we as mothers will still be considered the baby experts of the family. (He will most likely be thrilled to never own that title!) But we are partners in this whole parenthood deal, so let's act like it!

Partners, teammates, lovers, friends. There were a lot of terms to use when I thought about our couplehood. We'd been a couple for some time. We'd had a baby and proved a little something more to the world about the depth of our devotion. We'd more than just said vows in front of family and friends. We wildly and boldly meant them and spent as many commodities as it took to live them out.

So who were we becoming in all this? Who did we want to be?

A COUPLE OF PARENTS OR A COUPLE THAT PARENTS?

Were we going to settle on being a couple of parents, or could we actually become a couple *that* parents?

Dating after baby became essential. This didn't mean scheduling a regular babysitter or spending a lot of money on lavish dinners out. Frankly, that would have been fantastic but our resources didn't allow for that luxury, and that kind of expectation would have been too much.

What we lacked in resources we made up for in sincerity. I might cook him his favorite meal and we would wait until the baby fell asleep (mind you, this could be as late as 9 or 10 p.m. some nights) but we would stay up late and feast by ourselves in the comfort of our living room. Maybe he would change the baby one whole evening as I sipped a glass of wine, thankful that his heart for service was better than any bouquet of roses I could have ever received. Creativity and necessity tend to go hand in hand, but it's *keeping* the necessity for it that is the real purpose.

Babies demand a lot and often. But they grow, they change, they become ever more capable and unpredictable in what they require of you. Eventually they make their own value systems. Eventually they cash in their commodities for priorities of their own. And you are left staring at that other half of your couple, who will either recognize you or not. It all starts right now.

Marriage doesn't change; people do. The world changes. Ideas of love, concepts of success, even feelings of happiness all change. But marriage is and will always be the unified commitment to journey together along the same path toward the same goal. Marriage will always be the representation on Earth of how Christ loves His church.

WHAT BETTER INVESTMENT COULD YOU MAKE?

Falling in love with my husband is one of my favorite things to do. With each and every life change, I am given the opportunity to respond to God and my marriage with gratitude and to embrace the challenge of seeking selflessness through the power of the Holy Spirit. Besides, if that wasn't reason enough, it's wonderfully fun to get to know in a whole new way the person God selected for you as your teammate in this outrageous voyage called parenthood.

Just be careful. The more you get to know your husband, the more you might fall in love with him. The more you fall in love with your husband . . . well, I don't have to spell it out for you, but it probably led to what got you to pick up this book in the first place.

You Got This!

Dearest New Mama,

You got this. You were perfectly chosen by the King of Kings, the Ruler of the Universe, the Prince of Peace that surpasses all understanding to bear this new life. You got this! You were the perfect person, made wholly and solely to give birth to this child. Feel it, embrace it, own it. You got this.

You already love this baby more than anything you've ever loved before. You would do anything for this baby, and you are so beyond sure of that fact that it doesn't even matter what "anything" is . . . you're in. You can't comprehend your capacity for loving someone this much because it's never happened until now, and even still, after witnessing it for yourself, it doesn't feel real. You can't describe it with words. No picture can capture it. No song can resonate the feeling. No feeling can even contain the power of this immeasurable gift you've been given. It knows no bounds and is limitless in its expanse.

This is how God feels about you. Can you imagine it? In fact, you can't! Not even our wildest thoughts or notions come close to comprehending the vastness of His love, His grace, His truth, His compassion.

There is only one vital difference between your love for your child and God's love for you. God's love never fails. Better yet, it is incapable of failing. Equally, it is unchanging, and therefore steadfast in its perfection.

You, my dear, are going to make a hot mess of yourself as a parent. Your unbridled love and devotion to your child, your determination as a parent, your commitment as a mother—none of these can keep you from the challenges and obstacles and burdens that are to come. None of these will protect you from the frustration, worry, anger, resentment, guilt, or loneliness that motherhood will bring. It will all be worth it. You will be eternally grateful you've chosen this path in your life. But it's not without its difficulties or sorrows.

Moreover, you have just willingly doubled your chances for pain, as you gave up part of your heart to walk around the world outside of your body. Your child will forever affect you. Your child will forever impact you. For this, you are grateful and broken.

Fear not! Your mistakes will not be in vain, nor will your love. God will use it all. God doesn't love our sin, but He loves that our mistakes can be a constant reminder for how much we truly need Him, how we rarely know what to do, or how we continually choose our way over His. God loves when we turn to Him, seek Him out, cry to Him for help, pity, or justice. God wants you just as you want your child . . . regardless of motive, intention, or success. He will take you as you are, no matter what, no matter when.

You will do terrible things as a new mother. You will be confused and want to quit at some point. You may even have regrets or sabotage your own version of success by blaming any and every thing around you so you aren't at fault. It will suck. It will exhaust you. It will destroy you if you let it, and you will want to let it at times.

People will judge you as a mother. Some will give you terrible advice that won't work. Others will offer you comfort but only at the cost of feeling badly about yourself or admitting you should have known better. And your kid might not turn out the way you hoped. He or she might not believe what's true or fight for what's right. You might feel betrayed by all that you longed for. You might be left behind more broken than you began.

Still, God will be there. God will want you. God will love you. God will search for you and fight for you and hope for your best, just like you would for your child. Probably even more. Because God can't fail and God can't change and God can't stop loving you. Ever.

And, maybe, just maybe, even through all your trials and mistakes and the haphazard pandemonium we call parenthood, you still have a smile on your face. Perhaps you make it out alive and live to tell about it. Maybe your child even grows up to be a productive member of society or changes the world for the better. Maybe you will swell with pride and think it was all because of you, all the while keeping back the secret that you winged it just like the rest of the world. Even if you got the best advice from the wisest people and the encouragement of everyone in your community, you know in your heart you were merely the vessel who was privileged to witness such a success.

Still, God is there. Still, God is longing for you. Still, God pursues you. You have the same need for Him that you've always had. You, who owe it all to Him. You, who has a new baby that will need Him as well. You.

You got this. Because, my sweet one, He's got you.

~Pardymama

About the Author

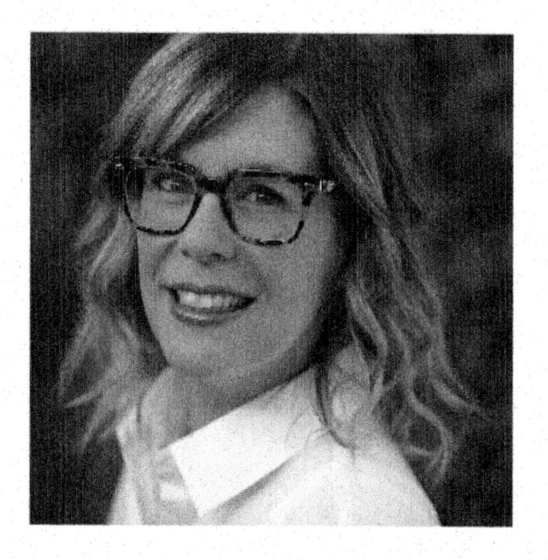

Emily Pardy is a thirty-something wife, mother of two, and full-time graduate student earning her masters degree in Marriage & Family Therapy. She has written for Thriving Family magazine, ParentLife magazine, Venn magazine, MOPs (Mothers of Preschoolers) and MOPs UK websites. She runs pardymama.com where she blogs regularly about motherhood, marriage, and other mayhem. Raising two daughters has taught her more about God, priorities, and her own vulnerability than anything else in life. Addicted to strong coffee and good conversation, she writes from her own experiences, unashamedly pulling back the curtain to reveal her personal thoughts and struggles for others to glean from. When she's not writing, she loves baking bread from scratch and playing dress up with her daughters. She lives with her husband and two girls in Nashville, Tennessee where they attend The Village Chapel.

CPSIA information can be obtained at www.ICGtesting.com
Printed in the USA
BVOW08s2028100515

399783BV00018B/440/P